To
a

Blessings & Joy
Linda Martin.

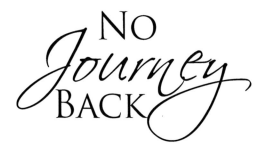

LINDA MARTIN

CROSSBOOKS

CrossBooks™
A Division of LifeWay
1663 Liberty Drive
Bloomington, IN 47403
www.crossbooks.com
Phone: 1-866-879-0502

Scripture taken from the New King James Version, Copyrighted 1979, 1980, 1982 By Thomas Nelson, Inc. Used by permission. All rights reserved.

©2011 Linda Martin. All rights reserved.

No part of this book may be reproduced, stored in a retrieval system, or transmitted by any means without the written permission of the author.

First published by CrossBooks 6/20/2011

Library of Congress Control Number: 2011930238

ISBN: 978-1-6150-7899-8 (sc)
ISBN: 978-1-6150-7900-1 (hc)

Printed in the United States of America

This book is printed on acid-free paper.

Any people depicted in stock imagery provided by Thinkstock are models, and such images are being used for illustrative purposes only.

Certain stock imagery © Thinkstock.

Because of the dynamic nature of the Internet, any web addresses or links contained in this book may have changed since publication and may no longer be valid. The views expressed in this work are solely those of the author and do not necessarily reflect the views of the publisher, and the publisher hereby disclaims any responsibility for them.

To Phillip, Angela, Randy,

Robin, Andy

And my precious grandchildren

May your journey in life be blessed

Acknowledgments

My deepest appreciation to the following people who helped in making this book possible:

Angela Martin Hale

Proof Reader

Suzanne Jamison

Technical and Design support

Michael Tuck

Photographic Assistance

My Encouragers

Those who prayed and stayed the journey with me to write this book

Contents

Acknowledgments	vii
Preface: No Journey Back	xi
Chapter 1: My Journey Begins	1
Chapter 2: Whose Am I?	11
Chapter 3: The Moth	15
Chapter 4: Healing Service	21
Chapter 5: The Rose	27
Chapter 6: Be a Witness	31
Chapter 7: Into Surgery	35
Chapter 8: God's Continuous Work	41
Chapter 9: Finger Paints	43
Chapter 10: Radioactive Treatment	47
Chapter 11: Moving On	51
Chapter 12: No Journey Back	55
Chapter 13: Generation to Generation	61
Chapter 14: The Blessing	65
Chapter 15: Family of God	69
Chapter 16: The Divided Sky	73
Chapter 17: Caught In the Act	77
Chapter 18: Santa Substitute	81
Chapter 19: The Stain	85
Chapter 20: The Doll	89
Chapter 21: Dyeing for the church	93
Chapter 22: The Borrowed Tree	97
Chapter 23: Miss Lucy	101
Chapter 24: The Table	105
Chapter 25: The Truth	109
Chapter 26: Beware of Job	113
Chapter 27: Uncle Raymond	117
Chapter 28: Letters	121
Chapter 29: Generations Come, Generations Go	125
Appendix	129
About the Author	139

Preface: No Journey Back

An old song says, "no turning back, no turning back." When my children were small, they loved to sit in "big church" and watch their daddy direct the music. As we sang that song, our daughter sang out in her loudest voice, "no journey back, no journey back." Her brother, Randy, would scream so everyone in the church could hear him that she "did it wrong again!" I would tell her the correct words, but it was no use. We all gave up on her. She would sing—and still does—with great enthusiasm, "no journey back, no journey back."

After weeks of seeking a title for this book, I found myself totally at a loss. I had prayed and prayed, but nothing seemed to come to me. Then as I lay in bed wide awake at 4:30 one morning, I reminded God that *we* had to find a title for this book. *We* were running out of time on our chosen date for completion. Strangely, for some reason, my mind went back to my children and my love for them. I thought about all I had endured with my cancer and about its effects on all of us. Suddenly I could hear Angela singing the "no journey back" song. I could see Randy punching her and letting her know that those were not the right words. I then knew the title of this book had to be *No Journey Back*.

I had begun a journey of no turning back when cancer came into my life. My journey started over two and one-half years ago with third-stage thyroid cancer. I cannot take a journey back in time far enough to catch the cancer before it formed in my body or before it progressed to stage three. I have learned a lot about myself and my family during my journey. I have learned so much more about my relationship with my God. He has been on this journey with me. He will not depart and He will never turn back from our journey together.

This book tells about my journey with cancer, but mostly about what awesome and great things God has done and is still doing in my life. I am indebted to so many friends and family members who have joined me in support and prayer on this journey. Indeed there will be *no journey back*. Life promises so much more to experience and to celebrate. What a wondrous journey is ahead for those of us who belong to Him. As the apostle writes, "…If you send them forward on their journey in a manner worthy of God you will do well" 3 John 1:6, (NKJV).

I pray I can, through this book, help you in your journey in a manner worthy of God, so that you and I will do and be well.

"No journey back, no journey back." Praise the Lord. Our *journey* lies ahead and God knows our destination. I look forward to arriving there to see my Savior and my God. Heaven awaits!

CHAPTER 1: *My Journey Begins*

My journey begins.

This week—I believe it was the last week of February or first part of March 2008—became a difficult week for me. I had been in Bluefield, West Virginia, the week before and had a terrible time with sinuses and an earache. In other words, a *yuck* week. I had gone to my family doctor and he said I had an ear infection in the right ear, as usual. He gave me a prescription for some medication. While there, I asked him to check the lump on the outside of my neck. I had seen him earlier and pointed it out to him. He had said not to worry about it, but we could watch it. This time I told him it was growing. Since I had first seen him, it had really grown in size. I could see it clearly when I swallowed. All I could think of was that my mother had died from non-Hodgkin's lymphoma. Her cancer had started with a lump on her neck.

He told me that he would set up an appointment as soon as possible for an ultrasound with *a specialist*. The appointment was set up quickly for Friday, March 8. The day came and I saw the doctor who did an ultrasound and a biopsy. All this was done without any numbing and—yes!—it really did hurt. Needles stuck into the neck are not very fun things, but *somehow* I made it through the procedure. I look back and realize that seeing all the small containers filled with fluid and whatever else was the grossest thing about the procedure.

I left the office and began my long days of waiting for the results. I was trusting God for a clear cancer-free report. I remember that my husband, Phillip, had a tough time waiting. I don't know many men who are patient when waiting. I had moments of wanting to run away and forget the past week or so, but I knew that I needed to be strong for him, so I could not break down and let go of the tears and fear. I prayed for God to give me the strength to endure. He came to my aid as usual.

Well, the waiting came to a halt very quickly. I was on the phone with my daughter, Angela, when a call came in on the other line. Angela, a high school English and Spanish teacher, was on her way to school. I told her to hold on while I checked the other line. It was the doctor's office asking if I could come in that morning. I told Angela that I needed to get off the line and go to the doctor's office at once.

Phillip and I quickly headed for the office, praying both for a good report and also for the tunnel traffic to be light. We wanted to get to the doctor's office almost instantly, but, on the other hand, we didn't want to get there at all. Our emotions were running faster than our car.

We arrived at the office and were shown to our room. The doctor came in almost at the same time we did. He sat down and pulled out the dreaded report. He was very soft-spoken in telling us that the test came back positive for cancer and we would need to see a surgeon as soon as possible. His office would call and set the appointment for me. I felt my blood turn to ice water, but I think I had already prepared myself for that report. I looked over at my husband and I knew he wanted to cry and to beg the doctor to change his words to say that the report showed no cancer. I felt so sorry for him, so I just asked God to give us both the strength we would need to go through all that would happen in the following days, weeks, and months.

After seeing the doctor, we decided to go by my husband's office, which was near the hospital and the doctor's office. Phillip was serving at a church in Virginia at that time. We walked into his office, trying to decide how we would tell the office staff the news we had just received. The staff members are such wonderful people and great prayer warriors (people dedicated to prayer). Before we could decide what to say, the pastor's secretary came by and saw us in the office. Her immediate question was "What are you two doing here today? It's your day off." We told her where we had been and about the results of the tests. Suddenly she reached out and put her hands on my neck and began praying for healing. It was such a spontaneous reaction I think I was as shocked as she was. She said that she really did not know what had come over her and that she had never done anything like that before.

She and I laughed, hugged one another, and then, with tears streaming down our faces, we walked from the office into the hallway. My husband was following behind us. We knew we looked "weird," because the receptionist stepped out of her office to see what was going on. We stopped and I shared with her my report concerning the cancer. She immediately hugged me tightly and began praying for healing. These two ladies, my friends, were so powerful in their prayers and love that I felt like a little chick being covered and protected by the wings of its mother. *How blessed my husband and I are,* I thought.

I knew from that moment that God had everything under His control. I would be loved, prayed for, and supported. On my journey, the ever-present Father, Son, and Holy Spirit would be right there with every step I took, even when I faced those steps that I sometimes thought that I could not take. If I needed to be carried, God would carry me; if I needed to cry, He would wipe away my tears; if I felt I could not carry the burden, He would carry it for me.

Within an hour, I found myself needing my tears wiped away and my torn heart mended as my phone rang and my husband answered with "Hello, son." My mother's heart was torn out to tell my son what I had just learned … We had not even had a chance to tell our daughter about the test results, but she had called our son Randy earlier to tell him that the doctor had called and asked us to come right in. She had put the old *two and two* together and called her brother. As I sat on our front porch in my white wicker rocking chair with a sweater wrapped around my trembling body, Phillip handed me the phone.

With every ounce of strength I had and all God would give me to keep my voice from breaking like my heart, I spoke. "Hello, my son …" Immediately I caught the tremble in Randy's voice. He really did not want to ask me the question weighing heavily on his heart, but I could sense his hesitation. I spoke first and asked how he was doing.

Randy was returning home from a business trip out of town. He lived in another state and for the first time I think he felt like he was on the other side of the world from me here in Virginia. He answered my question by saying, "I guess I am doing okay but how are things going with you and Dad?" He continued with a few sniffs, so I could tell he was holding back the tears. He said, "Angela called earlier and said you had to go see the doctor early this morning, so did you get your test results?"

I said, "Yes, son, I received the results." At that moment I really just wanted to stop the clock and call on Captain Kirk of the Starship *Enterprise* to say to Scotty, "Okay, Scotty, beam Linda over to her son Randy." I just wanted to be there to wipe away the tears that I knew were falling down his cheeks. I wanted to hold him like the times when he was a little boy and had a bad "boo boo"; to tell him everything was fine, but now he is an adult and I would need him to dry my tears and give me the hug and tell me, "Yes, Mom, everything will be just fine."

My mind flashed back to the various times in Randy's life and challenges he had faced. One was when he was about two months old. I was giving him his midmorning bath when I sensed something was wrong with him. I noticed he was his usual jolly self by splashing water everywhere. He looked and acted perfectly normal, but I could not overcome this feeling that something was wrong. I lifted him out of the tub, wrapped him in a big towel, and held him close to me. Finally I decided to call our friend and pediatrician who took care of Randy and his older sister, Angela. "Doc" told me that he had a break in appointments so I could bring Randy in and he would check him over. I quickly put the kids into the car and rushed to his office. He came into the room and remarked that Randy sure looked fine. In fact, he had seen him at church a few days earlier and all seemed well. Doc had checked the usual ears, throat, etc. but when he put the stethoscope up to Randy's chest he held it there for longer than usual. I knew something was wrong. He turned and spoke with urgency in his voice for me to get Randy next door to the hospital immediately. He called out to his nurse to call the hospital and tell them to get Randy admitted and in oxygen at once. He would be right over to check on him. I became terrified when I heard those words, but I knew to follow his orders. Somewhere I managed to call my husband at church and he rushed to the hospital. That began a long week of intense treatment for pneumonia for our young baby boy. He was so bad we could not get him out and hold him or feed him. The chance of losing him tore at my heart. It was at that moment that I realized I needed to turn him over to God. Little did I know just how many times and battles would be ahead for me to give to God. Prayer became as important to me as breathing, and I would teach my children to have faith in prayer to our God.

Randy would find out by experience when he was about sixteen just how prayer could get him through all stages of life. When he was a young boy, he loved airplanes (and still does). He and his dad spent days upon days at the airport where they watched planes. His teachers would tell us that when a plane went over the school building, they would have to stop class while Randy told the class what type plane was flying and all its stats. He had taken flying lessons and now it was time for his big test for his license. He came home one afternoon and began telling me that he didn't think he could pass the test. He began to get all emotional and feel quite defeated, ready to give it all up. I turned to him and asked him *who* made him. Just as Randy started to answer, I anticipated his answer and told him not to say that Mom and Dad made him. He looked at me and replied that God had made him. I then told Randy to always remember that since God had made him, God should be the one to give him his limitations in life. He should always do his best, praying and trusting God for all things. Randy had been sitting on the bed during our conversation, so he stood up, walked over to his desk, picked up his books, and began studying. The next day he took the test and passed. Flying became an important part of Randy's life for many years.

Now, as I sat on my porch listening to him and how my son had grown in the Lord, I did indeed realize that my message to him had come full circle back to me. God had made me and now God should be the one putting limitations on my life. It was my job to trust Him in all things and in all ways. With prayer on my lips and thankfulness for Randy, I realized it was time for me to say, "The results were positive for thyroid cancer." I gave him all the information we had at the moment. His reply was so unexpected that I had to laugh when he said that he was in the car driving home when his sister called. She said she just knew that the report had to be positive for cancer since the doctor wanted me in his office immediately. Randy said, "I really knew then that it had to be bad, so I got so mad at God that I yelled at Him. I put the car window down and took my round tin of Skoal chewing tobacco into my hand and threw it out the car window as hard as I could."

Well, I laughed because I truly doubted Randy would do such a thing. I probably had misunderstood him because he was a former police officer and a fanatic about people throwing things out of cars. I was suddenly brought back to reality when I heard him saying that I had always been the one who ate right and never smoked, and now I am the one with cancer. He continued, "It just isn't right. There are too many other bad, mean, and ungodly people who should have this, not you."

I really appreciated his honesty because I guess I had had those same thoughts. But then I realized that many times I have heard that it rains on the just and unjust alike.

Matthew 5:45 says, *"...And sends rain on the just and on the unjust"* (NKJV).

Oh, but what God had in store for me! That is what will make me be obedient to God and write why it *rained* on me that day and what God has done and is still doing in my life. I just hope it will bring strength to others as I have been strengthened. Well, back to Randy and his outburst. I still laugh when I think of what would have happened if indeed he did throw out that tobacco can and it hit a police car. How would Randy have explained a flying can of Skoal? At times even today, when our family is having a rough day or situation, we laugh and say that it's a "throw out the can of Skoal" day.

We talked for a few more minutes and then I asked him not to call his sister but wait for us to give her a call when she got out of school. I don't know if Randy called her or not, but we assured him we would keep him updated daily and that we loved him. Next would be to call his sister, because I knew they would need each other during this time.

Why is it that, when you think you have all your emotions under control, you realize you were just kidding yourself? That is what happened when I hung up the phone after talking with Randy. Angela called and wanted to know what had happened at the doctor's office. It again was hard to talk with her even though she was only about six hours from us—it was still separation. I took a deep breath and repeated the same words that I had shared with Randy. She had lots of questions as well and wanted to know if she should come up to be with us or what she could do. I told her that we were to see a surgeon and probably have more tests before getting a surgery date. Angela is the type of person who often can control her emotions when she really needs to, but she will let it all go later. I could tell that this was the situation now. I knew she would have her "throw out the can of Skoal" time later. I assured her we would be fine and would let her know as soon as we received any more information. Later, Angela shared with me that, after our talk on the phone, she took a long walk down the country road where she lives. She said she prayed and told Satan to take his hands off me. Then she "reminded" God of my years of service to Him and His responsibility to protect me.

Angela's words of "God's responsibility to protect me" seemed strange at first. I suddenly remembered that those were words I had spoken about her before she was born. My husband and I were married for about six years before I became pregnant. We had wanted children but had about given up on conceiving. We had begun discussing adoption and were considering adopting a young child instead of a baby. We felt there were so many young children who needed a home. Well, one day, what I thought was a reaction to some general medication turned out to be the great news that I was pregnant! We were thrilled and our parents could not believe it. This would be the first grandchild for my parents who were beyond joyful. But, a few weeks after our great news, I was talking with a lady I knew and holding her son when she remarked that the doctor had said he thought the boy had German measles. I could not believe that I was exposed to that disease. Then I remembered that I had also had a radioactive scan about the same time I became pregnant. With these two situations, I almost fell apart. The doctor explained what could happen if I carried the baby after being exposed to these things. I knew that deformities and other problems could occur with the baby as well as miscarriage. Never for one moment would we consider any options but to put our trust in our God who had created this child. We would trust Him to the birth, care, and protection of this wonderful answer to our prayers.

Praise be to God that Angela was born a few weeks early and in perfect health. In fact, you would have had a hard time proving to us that she was not the most beautiful baby born that day.

Angela continued to grow and be in great health until suddenly, at about age nine, a health issue developed and would go on for a long time. She appeared to be the perfect picture of health, but we and the doctors knew something was wrong. She began many stays in the hospital. One particular time, after a test, the doctor called me to give me an update. My husband had gone to the airport miles away from our house when the call came in. I needed to reach him, but, since he had no cell phone, I had to call the airport to have him paged. I finally reached him on the phone and told him to get home at once. I told him the doctor wanted Angela in the hospital immediately.

He rushed home and, as we were packing her bag, Randy walked in and looked at us. Frightened, he asked us if his sister was going to die. Our hearts and time seemed to stop. True, we had had those thoughts during all these hospital visits, but we were staying strong in our faith for her healing. Each time Angela would go into the hospital, I would assure her that God would protect her and be with her. Finally a day came when one specialist came out of his office after examining her and said he had to ask us a question about our heritage. He explained that there was a disease that was more prevalent in certain nationalities. He asked if either one of us was of Italian heritage. My husband replied that he was Italian. His dad is full Italian. The doctor said that he hated to ask the next question, but it was important. His question was if both or either grandparents were from Sicily. My husband turned very pale and very quietly answered that his grandmother was from Sicily. The doctor looked at us but did not say a word for a few moments. Then he explained that he was going to do a blood test for a certain disease and a positive for the disease would not be a good result. (After all these years I feel confident this disease has been conquered.) Anyway, we had to wait for a week or longer for the results since the test had to be sent out of state to a special lab.

There was a lot of prayer during this time and affirmation to Angela that God's protective hand was upon her and us as her family. He would give us peace. The day the phone rang and the nurse told us that the doctor wanted to see us was finally here. We went to the office and sat down awaiting and preparing for what the lab had found. In a few minutes, the doctor came in and explained that the blood test revealed that all was clear. She did not have the disease. He did let us know that he had done all he could for her, but he had recommended that she be accepted into a university hospital study and be under their care.

We were moving in that direction when her problem stopped just as suddenly as it had started. We kept in touch with the doctor, but, to this day, she has been healed.

Indeed, she knew all about how to give me comfort at my time of facing cancer again. It is so amazing how much my children have grown in the Lord and I had a real comfort that, when they went to God in prayer, He would hear them. I knew that, as I prayed for them, they would be comforted. My children have always had loving and giving hearts. It was hard to imagine now in these days that they would be my strength, giving me the hugs for my big "boo boo" of cancer. Randy, Angela, and their dad would be God's angels here on earth to take care of me, to comfort me, and to lift me up in prayer every day.

I am so blessed, I thought. I have just finished talking to my two children while sitting here on my front porch. I looked over at my husband sitting in his white wicker chair and saw the tiny tears in his eyes. His big black eyebrows were moving up and down, and I can always tell that he is in deep thought when he does that. I looked away and stifled my giggle, turning to ask him just what he was so deep in thought about. He looked at me and gave me a big grin and I knew he has been replaying all that had happened this day. He was thinking about how strong our family is and how fortunate we all are to belong to God. God will take care of us all and everything will be just fine. Yes, it will.

CHAPTER 2: *Whose Am I?*

Who do I belong to? As a Christian, that has always been an easy answer. I belong to God. But have you ever been face to face with someone who tried to prove that you were just kidding yourself? How secure are you really in God's hands? My reassurance came in a very unexpected way, one that I hope I never have to go through again but am glad I experienced.

At this point, I wrestled with just how to present this unique and somewhat shocking experience. Some may question if I was truly awake or just having a dream. I must assure you that every detail was real and I was fully awake. First let me share a Scripture verse, which I realize we don't often take truly to heart and mind.

1 Peter 5:8: "Be sober, be vigilant; because your adversary the devil walks about like a roaring lion, seeking whom he may devour" (NKJV).

Satan is the master of disguise. There was the time when I was visiting my daughter who lived in another city. We had gotten up early to go to breakfast together at one of *America's favorite restaurants*. We stepped up to the crowded counter and placed our order. I gave the clerk a ten-dollar bill. I quickly realized she had not given me the correct change so I asked if she would check her drawer to see what I had given her. She emphasized the amount I had given her and told me that she had given me the correct change. She replied that she could not open her drawer to check. The manager came up and asked if there was a problem. She opened the drawer. Everyone watched the situation develop as the manager said in a somewhat loud voice that I had given the clerk a ten-dollar bill. I explained that was correct but she had given me change for twenty dollars. I told her I was a Christian and I could have pocketed the money, but that was not what God would have wanted me to do. What if I kept the money and someone in the crowd knew me and saw what I had done? Lying and stealing are not what a Christian should do. The manager stood speechless for a moment, then took the change and apologized along with giving us extra food. I thanked her and turned around to come face to face with a pastor I knew standing along with people from a local church. So you see, Satan disguised himself in the form of money in the hope that I would sell my witness for a few dollars.

It was a very simple disguise most of us have been a part of, but so many times it has been the roaring lion disguise we may recognize first. What I found out is that Satan will go to any extreme to devour us. He wants to destroy and capture our souls and to give us doubts about our relationship with God. I had no idea that he was walking around my house one night hoping to devour me and my faith in my God. I had no knowledge what and who I was about to come face to face with in just a few hours.

A few days after the cancer diagnosis, Phillip and I were finally able to go to bed at a reasonable hour. We got into bed, talked a while, and then prayed for God's continued care for us and for the healing of my body. I continued to pray silently as I fell asleep. Suddenly I was awakened by the feeling that someone was in our bedroom. I could feel my husband beside me and was about to wake him up when my eyes were drawn to the foot of the bed. There, standing at the foot of the bed, was something I could not believe, something that was so grotesque that I could not help but stare. That alone was a surprise to me that I could stare at this *creature* instead of screaming and crawling over my husband to get out of the room or, better yet, out of the house. I have to admit that I am not the world's bravest woman. I was looking at this being when suddenly he turned his head and looked at me …

I say *he* because its upper body had the very masculine appearance of a man. I knew this, yet he did not really look like a man. Its shape was formed by a mixture of drab grays with very small amounts of dirty white. Its head seemed to be too heavy for its body. It had no eyes or nose as such, but I knew it could see and hear. I did not see normal ears. The head was totally barren of any normal human features.

It had long arms that were slender from elbow to wrist. The hands were very large and the fingers were large and all the same length. The right side of the hip area was shaped like a horse's hip all the way down to the beginning of the knee area.

I have to say that, at the time everything was happening, I knew every single detail of this form, but, after being made fully aware of it, I *felt* that I was not to know everything concerning whatever this was.

I saw the creature *look* startled. (Remember, it had no normal face, but I knew it had emotions that showed a startled reflex.) It walked very fast toward my husband's bedroom closet. I saw the closet door open but knew it was closed when we went to bed. My husband and I don't like the door open, because if we get up at night we can run into it. "Why is the door open?" I asked myself. I knew there was something that the creature heard to cause it to hurry toward the closet.

As it approached the closet, it began to curl its shoulders and lower its head into its hands. It cowered when a voice from the closet area said, "You cannot hide from me. You know that." The *voice* was strong and firm, but for some reason I was not as afraid of this voice as the creature seemed to be. There were words from the creature and then words almost like an argument developed between the two. Suddenly there was the appearance of two hands from the *good* voice that I knew. These hands were of a color I can't explain—not gold, bronze, or yellow but yet a color. They were very large and hovered around the creature's torso. Suddenly the right hand of the good one snatched the entire torso of the creature. One hand completely surrounded the torso of the creature. The voice of the good one said, "Satan, you cannot have her." I felt the voice of the good one say to the creature that he could not snatch me from His hands. I knew all this was just between me, the good one, and Satan because my husband was still asleep beside me. I felt the presence of the Holy Spirit, God, look at me, and we began to talk. It was so wonderful. He is the most trusted one I have ever known. A real calm peace and contentment filled me and not for one second did I have fear, not even from the very beginning of this encounter.

I felt someone shaking me and realized it was my husband asking me if I was okay. I did not want to answer him and interrupt my conversation with God. The shaking continued and I finally had to answer him. I replied that yes, I was fine. I was only talking with God. It was just as if I had been talking to a dear friend forever. I felt such a peace but missed finishing the conversation with God. I don't remember anything we talked about, but I felt total contentment.

A few days later, Phillip and I were in the car and I asked him again why he had disturbed me. He said, "I thought you were having a nightmare." I asked him why he thought that. He explained that I wasn't screaming or thrashing about or anything weird, except talking. I asked him why he would consider my talking a nightmare. His answer shocked me. He replied that I was speaking in a language that was beautiful, but one that he had never heard before. It was a language that he could not understand or even begin to explain. He said he could not get over its beauty. I knew that I understood everything God was telling me and I assumed that I was speaking in English to God as I always did. My husband's remarks amazed me. I had never before or after that night spoken in any other language when talking with God. Naturally, having served in a Spanish-speaking country as a missionary, I spoke Spanish, but so does my husband. He would have understood that language. I just accepted that for some reason I may never know here on earth why perhaps God chose for me to speak to Him that way. As I said, I could not give a detailed description of what our conversation was, but, every once and a while when I am praying or resting in His comfort, I have feelings of His complete presence with me. I wish I could find the words to write, but I strive in vain. I only praise Him for His many wonderful works in my life.

The next day my husband and I opened the Bible to have our devotion. We were led to the tenth chapter of John. We began reading and soon realized why God had led us to that chapter. It was the confirmation of what had happened. We read the following:

John 10:27–30: "My sheep hear My voice, and I know them, and they follow Me. And I give them eternal life, and they shall never perish; neither shall anyone snatch them out of My hand. My Father, who has given them to Me, is greater than all; and no one is able to snatch them out of My Father's hand. I and My Father are one" (NKJV).

CHAPTER 3: *The Moth*

I am an "early riser," usually waking up around 5:00 a.m., so I use this time for Bible study and prayer. I will get up and go to another room and begin my day with God. If I felt I would disturb my husband, I would just lie in bed and use the quiet time to pray—to talk with God. This particular morning, I prayed about the cancer surgery that was coming up soon. I had already been praying for healing as well as having others praying for me. As I lay there, I made my request known to God. I had a heavy heart knowing just what cancer can do, not only to the "victim," as some would say, but also to family and even friends. In fact, when you mention to a stranger that you have cancer, they will sometimes look like you have a contagious disease and they want to run from you as fast as they can. Cancer does come with a stigma. I thought about my children, my husband, my brothers, and oh so many people who are so special to me. I remembered my mom and other family members who had passed on as the result of cancer.

I felt the tears fall from my eyes as I shared my heart with God and my desire to be healed from this disease. I want to live to see my children grow old and experience the beauty of being grandparents. I want to see my grandchildren graduate from high school and college, to attend their weddings, and to be there when my great-grandchildren are born. I still had so many things I wanted to do for God and, through Him, accomplish what He has in store for me. I love sharing Jesus and the plan of salvation with others and I wanted to have years left to be His witness. I thought of my husband and how alone he would feel. We have been together so many years and I just could not begin to think of him leaving me. How would he feel as he stood beside the casket at the graveside? What intimate things would he whisper to me? What would be the regrets, the joys, the desires of his heart, the things he had wanted to do with me but could not do now? Oh, so many things rushed through my mind!

I finally got control of my emotions and felt the pillow now wet with tears, tears not so much for myself but for others. I silently cried out to God to give me strength and especially to heal my body. I began to pray and found myself searching for words to express my desire for healing. Then I said, "God, I want you to heal my body, just like, just like …" I thought for a few seconds and suddenly the picture of a closet filled with clothes and a big, beautiful moth flying around the clothes looking for a garment from which to take a big bite came to me. "God," I said, "I want you to heal the cancer just like the moth eats clothes. Eat the cancer out of me, and, dear God, just as a moth will eat the cashmere clothes he likes best, you eat the cancer from me just like a cashmere garment. I want it all gone."

I was so excited about coming up with that analogy that I got up out of bed and felt so great. Well, guess what? I began to open my Bible to read a passage I felt I was led to in the Old Testament: Psalm 51. I turned to that passage and began to read, but shortly I realized that did not sound like Psalm 51 so I looked at the top of the page of the Bible and it said Isaiah 51. I again thought that was weird, so I started to turn back to Psalm 51. How could I make this mistake of getting these two books confused? I felt an urging to stay where I was reading and not to turn back to Psalm 51. I thought I would follow this urging and continue to read in Isaiah 51. Why? I don't know. Then I came upon Isaiah 51:8: "For the moth will eat them up like a garment, and the worm will eat them like wool; but my righteousness will be forever and my salvation from generation to generation" (NKJV).

When I finished reading this Scripture, I thanked God for giving me a good laugh at myself. I had been so smug to think I had come up with that analogy of the moth and garment. He knew just how to put me in my place! I really thanked Him for that. I turned back to finish reading the chapter. I closed my study with praise, thanksgiving, and my claim of the cancer to be eaten up from my body so I could see generation after generation of my family come to salvation and blessings in my dear Savior.

I could hardly wait for the time to pass until I could call Phillip's sister who lived in another town. We were never very close until her mother (my dear mother-in-law) passed away. I am amazed that we have become so close now, which I would never have imagined. I began to reminisce about the first time I met Norma. I lay down on the sofa and let the thoughts take me back to a special event in my life; a time that I would be meeting my future in-laws and family. Phillip and I had just become engaged and he was taking my mother and me to meet his family who lived about six hours from us. We had set out on our journey early one beautiful morning, stopping along the way for lunch, and later for Mom and me to freshen up before arriving at the Martins' home.

I think we all had a moment of panic, asking ourselves the usual questions about whether we would like each other, etc. Well, we arrived shortly before dinner and went to sit on the front porch. I liked being out in the open since I thought I could escape if we needed to make a quick escape. Mother-in-law stories rambled about in my mind. Talk began about the wedding: when, where, time, and, of course, my gown, which I still did not have. Time passed rather quickly and soon we were sitting down to dinner. Mother and I ate sparingly. We were nervous and a bit scared about staying in the country. (At the time, it looked like country to us, but later I realized it was just the suburbs.) We had heard all the stories about the bears that would come down from the national forest just above their home and we certainly did not like spending the night in bear country. One terrifying thought that came into our minds was the fact that we would need to walk out back to the "facilities." Phillip's dad had built their home but had not completed the bathroom. He worked in Washington, DC, as a carpenter and did great work. The house was wonderful, except for that delay in the building process.

After dinner, Dorothy (my future mother-in-law) and Mother went into the living room to sit and visit but, unknown to anyone else Mother had told me she needed to have a cigarette. She had asked me if I would go to the outhouse with her so she could smoke. I could see she was as nervous as a cat on a hot tin roof. I had to do something. I went into the kitchen to find Phillip and whispered to him the dilemma Mother was in. I told him she would have a nicotine fit if I didn't get her out soon. He told me to come with him. We walked into the living room and Phillip looked at his mother and told her that my mom was craving a cigarette. I thought Mother was going to faint with embarrassment. His mom jumped up from her chair and turned to my mother. It scared me and I thought we would be thrown out of the house. To my shock, she asked my mom if she had any cigarettes because, if she didn't, she had plenty and was "dying to have a smoke." I was thrilled I would not have to travel the path out back to the outhouse or be outside in bear country. Well, from that moment on there was a bond between those two that lasted a lifetime.

I would not want to lead anyone to believe that I was happy with their smoking. Years later, my mother would suffer from throat cancer and pass away from another form of cancer. Phillip's mom also developed health problems.

My first meeting with my mother-in-law was one of love for her. I treasured her love for me and she was a dear friend. I never had any negative mother-in-law stories to tell about her.

Norma and I always tolerated each other, though. In fact, I think we would avoid each other, but to this day we have no reason or understanding why we were so distant. I would tell Phillip each time we were to visit that I hoped Norma wasn't home, and, as I learned years later, she would ask her mother if she had to be around me. As the years passed, we managed to be kind and courteous to one another, but there was no real love. I honestly never gave it much thought, but just accepted our relationship.

The call about his mom came from Phillip's family late one evening. We had gone to visit her in the hospital earlier, but now she was home and not doing well. We were planning to go to see her the next day, not realizing she would not make it through the next day. The second call came very early the next morning. His mom and my precious mother-in-law was now with Jesus. Phillip had great comfort in the knowledge that both his mother and father had accepted the Lord as their Savior, even so late in life. He had the great honor of baptizing them both. My thoughts now turned to how Norma would feel toward me. I knew her pain was great, because losing a mother is like losing a part of your life. I began praying for her and the family. We both had suffered in the loss of a precious person in our lives and I had to let Norma know that.

Would she reject me, react in anger toward me in her hurt? I would soon find out.

Phillip and I left to travel to his mom's house shortly after that early call letting us know that his mom had gone into the arms of Jesus. We arrived later in the day and began that seemingly long walk from the car into the house. When we walked into the house, Norma immediately reached to hug him. I pulled him from her and grabbed her with tears running down my cheeks. Something happened at that moment, a bonding that made us closer than blood sisters. From that day on, we have shared all things with each other, especially spiritual matters. This prayer and Scripture concerning the moth had to be shared with her. I was so excited to hear her thoughts about the Scripture and affirmation concerning my healing. Well, the hour finally came when I knew she would be *up and about* as we would say. I dialed the phone, still trying to believe what had happened just a few hours ago. The phone rang several times and I began to think about what I would do if she didn't answer. How could I contain this within me? Just then she picked up the phone and I told her just about word for word what had happened to me that morning.

She said to wait just a minute because she had to get her Bible to see how her version read. I held the phone for what seemed like forever but in fact was just a minute. I was still in that almost unbelieving state of what had really happened. Norma answered the phone with a very shaky voice. I thought she sounded like she had been running. I knew she kept her Bible close by on the table, so why did she sound so out of breath? What had happened to her? She began to speak and I could hardly believe what she was saying to me. She said, "Linda, when I picked up my Bible, it fell open to Isaiah 51!" Norma told me that she had put a church bulletin in her Bible at random. She never put anything like that in her Bible and left it there. I was now in a state of complete awe. With almost no voice at all, Norma told me that she was stunned. I asked her what the date was on the bulletin and she said it was from Easter Sunday. Out of curiosity, I asked her what the pastor had preached on that Sunday. She answered that he had preached from Ephesians 3:20: "Now to him who is able to do exceedingly abundantly above all that we ask or think, according to the power that works in us."

Ephesians 3:21 says, "To Him be glory in the church by Christ Jesus to all generations, forever and ever. Amen" (NKJV).

Together we both, over the phone, laid claim to the healing of God upon my body that I am and will forever be cancer-free. I will live to see my children become grandparents, my great-grandchildren born, my husband and I will grow old together, and, most of all, I will see generations come to the Lord.

I believe He will use this book to be a witness to Him, His healing power, and His glory.

CHAPTER 4: *Healing Service*

I had already begun to pray about my healing and others were praying for me as well. I began to spend more time in Scripture reading about healing. Perhaps I was so thirsty to know more about healing it was like being in a desert searching for water. I would find *healing* messages from so many sources, as well as from the Bible. I recall having the television on one morning and just as I was about to change the channel the priest who was conducting a service said, "I believe there is someone with thyroid cancer who needs special prayer for healing today." I was somewhat surprised to hear that, but I stopped and accepted that prayer of healing from him. Sometime later I again turned the television on and a minister from a different faith was saying that he felt a need to pray for a lady that had just learned she had thyroid cancer, and he began praying. I again stopped and accepted that prayer.

I thought that God was really a God of humor but still worked in a mysterious way to reaffirm me in my prayer of healing. It came in the form of an egg. Our family was with us one morning when I opened a carton of eggs. I picked one egg up and to my *shock* there was an egg with a mark on it that looked like a cross, and in bright pink I might add. Now I really began to get the message that God was indeed still in charge of my life, and He was giving me affirmation in many ways as to His power of healing.

The time came for God to work in my pastor's heart to have a healing service at our church. My husband told me that the pastor would like to have the service on a Sunday night and wanted to know if

I would participate. I knew God was again making sure that I knew He was still in control of my life and was using so many people to reaffirm me of being healed.

As I began thinking about the upcoming service, I recalled the first time I had seen anyone healed. It just so happened that I would be a small part of this service. I grew up in a small coal-mining town in Virginia. We had a company store, school, and two churches. One church was for the "white" folk and the other was for the "colored" folk. That was something I could never quite understand. We had so many nationalities—Polish, Hungarian, and German—that it always confused me as to how one determined color of skin. Most all of the coal miners looked dark to me, so why did most of them go to the "white" church? My best friend was Carol Sue and she was "colored." I thought she was beautiful. Often after church on Sunday I would sneak off to her house and we would eat tomatoes from a can. I loved to stand outside their church and listen to their service. Sometimes I would get brave and peek in a window. They seemed to be having more fun than us white folks. Oh, we would have shouting, or "getting happy" as it was commonly called. There were foot washings and long-winded preachers—sometimes three or four a night. But most important, and what impressed me most with both churches, was prayer. I was almost afraid to go inside the church during prayer because I really expected to see God appear in the small room. When prayer for the sick was said, you really expected to see them recover quickly.

I was about six or seven when I found my grandfather in bed sick. I was so scared because I loved him so very, very much. I would get up early every day even when school was out. I would run up the road—we didn't have sidewalks—to my grandparents' house. All the houses were similar with four rooms, a screened porch off the kitchen, and a big front porch. We all had outhouses and a big round tub for Saturday night baths. Most of the coal miners used a large boarding/bathhouse for their showers after work. Well, on this particular morning, I ran into Ma's house expecting to see my Pa sitting at the kitchen table drinking his coffee from a saucer. I could hardly wait for us to go for a walk. When I walked into the kitchen, I could feel the heat from the old coal-burning stove so I stepped around it to see my Ma on the kitchen porch. I then saw my Pa in the big old iron bed that was kept on the kitchen porch in the summer. Ma looked at me and told me that Pa was sick. I was terrified because I had never seen him in bed after 6:00 a.m. I was scared because I did not really know what was wrong with him. My grandmother told me to run and get some of the elders of the church and bring them to the house at once. She said, "Tell them Charlie needs them."

I took off with my little skinny legs going as fast as they could. I would hit the gravel on the road and slide, but nothing would keep me from my job. I found one man in his yard and yelled to him, another working on a car, and two more talking to each other. When I yelled to them that Charlie needed them, they dropped what they were doing and ran with me to the house. I rushed back in time to see my Pa getting out of bed. The men gathered around my grandfather as he knelt on the floor. They laid their hands on him and began to pray. Sometime later, after what I thought was a long, long prayer, he got up and shook their hands as they left. He then went in and changed clothes, ate breakfast and, most of all, he drank his coffee from his saucer. Those prayers were heard and God had healed my grandfather. That image has stayed in my mind for all these years for just this time for reassurance of how great my God is—a God who is the same today as yesterday and is in the future. I needed him in the *now*.

The night of our healing service came and the church was excited. Our pastor began the healing service by asking if I would come up first and be seated in one of the chairs that had been arranged for the healing service. Then he asked for anyone else who wanted to be prayed for to please come and be seated with me at the front of the sanctuary. About nine others came forward, including a young man who had gone through thyroid cancer surgery sometime earlier. He came and sat down beside me. Then the pastor asked the deacons to please come forward to stand near us. He explained about the anointing of the oil as he placed it on each of our foreheads. He then asked the deacons to please take our hands into theirs and for those standing in back of us to place their hands on our shoulders. One man took my entire right hand into his while another took just the fingers of my left hand into his hand. I glanced back and saw my husband standing behind me with his hands on my shoulders.

The pastor began to pray. He had prayed a couple of sentences when I suddenly felt someone slip their fingers into the palm of my left hand. The hand felt so soft, like silk floating down, and I became startled asking myself who this could be. How could a person get this close to hold my hand? Then, without a bit of warning, a terrible pain hit the area of the throat where the growth was located. I prayed along with the pastor and asked that Satan be rebuked and leave me alone. The pastor continued in his prayer and I could feel the presence of the Holy Spirit when, suddenly, the hand that was holding my left hand pressed very firmly into the center of my palm. I was totally unaware of anyone else except the *new* hand that was touching me. Then the pain immediately left me. Suddenly, just as quickly as it had appeared, the hand disappeared from my hand just as the pastor was closing his prayer. I immediately looked up but did not see anyone else who had joined our group. We were all in the same position as when we began except we now had tears in our eyes. It was as if no one wanted to move. The presence of the Holy Spirit was so great.

A few days later, I asked my husband who the person was that had come into the group and placed his hand into the palm of my hand. He said he had not seen anyone else come into the group, but I explained to him what had happened. The next day, he mentioned it to the pastor and the pastor said that no else had come into the group near me. The two men who held my hands were questioned but again said no one else was there. They said if anyone had come, it would have caused everyone to shift position because we were so crowded into the space.

A little later, I again asked my husband if he would get the names of the men holding my hands, especially the name of the third person. I wanted to send them a thank-you note. I was totally unaware that my husband had already asked about the third person. He said he had not found out who it was. The next day a friend called and asked me to tell her about the third hand. I asked her what she was talking about and she said she had heard someone say that I wanted to know who it was. I said yes, I did want to know this person, and I told her the story as I have written it here. She then told me of a conversation between the pastor and the two men, her husband being one of the men holding my hand. Her husband had said shortly after the prayer, but before closing, something electrifying passed through their hands. People had been commenting on the moving of the Holy Spirit in the service. Their unanimous conclusion was that the third hand was none other than the hand of the Lord Himself.

CHAPTER 5: *The Rose*

We had experienced a great healing service and it was hard to get back to the reality of what we were still to face. My husband was busy making travel arrangements for our son and family. We were excited that they were coming to be with us. A special treat was to see our grandchildren. We had worked hard taking care of small tasks and needed a break. My husband suggested that we get out of the house and go for a drive. We drove out to one of our favorite places, a nearby park. It was a beautiful, quiet place on the bay. We loved to watch the small boats with the fishermen casting their lines far into the deep water. Sometimes a large boat would come along and the small boats would rock like they were going to turn over. It was funny to see the fishermen try to keep their balance in the wake left by the large boats.

We watched as large commercial ships passed by and we played guessing games as to what they contained within their hulls. Often we would see large navy ships and wonder what place they would be going to next or where they had been. How many people would the ship hold? All sorts of guessing games would play in our heads. Often we would stop and buy or bring our lunch or dinner to eat in the car by the bay. We sometimes stopped by the ice-cream store where I would get a big walnut sundae and Phillip would get a large cone of vanilla ice cream. We felt like newlyweds on a shoestring budget. Don't splurge on real food, just splurge on ice cream. We laughed again and again over silly things we had done, but now, at this stage of our lives, we shed a few tears. Suddenly we realized we were sitting there not making a sound and all the world seemed to be silent as we were mesmerized by the big beautiful red, orange, and golden sun as it began to slide into the distant ocean connected to the bay water. My husband gently reached over and held my hand as the sun dipped lower behind the water and began to disappear from our sight. It was time to go home.

A few days passed and my surgery was now upon me. I had done as most women would do: I made sure the house was cleaned; clothes were washed and ironed; and the refrigerator was cleaned and well-stocked with my family's favorite goodies. I then did what I really had been postponing and that was packing for my hospital stay. I asked myself if I needed a gown and pajamas, and what about shampoo and cosmetics? Did I have my favorite Bible set aside to be packed? But the truth was that I really knew I was just delaying the inevitable. I threw some items into the small suitcase and told my husband that if I needed anything else he could get the items from this drawer or that drawer. Now everything was done and I began waiting for the words, "It's a *go!*"

Late afternoon arrived so quickly and I found myself alone and thinking about what I had been told about the surgery and some things that could happen. One major concern was, because of the location of the cancer, it was possible that my vocal chords could be damaged. I thought about the many precious people I had known throughout the years who could not speak and how they used sign language to communicate. I had at one time taken a sign-language class taught by a couple who used signing as their primary means of communicating since they were limited in vocal communication. I had, just a few months ago, given away most of my signing books and had forgotten the majority of the signing skills I had learned. Now I wondered if I would need to learn signing again. Yes, of course there was concern about losing use of my vocal chords. I finally realized that I was spending too much time worrying about things that I had already turned over to God. If I lost my voice or the cancer had spread or so if something else happened during surgery, it was not in my power to change. I claimed God's healing hand upon my body and I had to leave the outcome with Him.

Sometime later, my husband came into the room and told me that we needed to go out for a few things. I grabbed my purse and shoes (I always go barefoot in the house) and we walked out to the van. I remembered that I had left a book on the back seat that I wanted to take with me to the hospital. I opened the back door of the van and a sweet aroma of roses rushed out to greet me. I stepped back and glanced around to see what was causing the rose aroma when I spotted a rose bush on the floor. Phillip asked me what was wrong so I asked what he was doing with a rose bush in the van. His face became a bright shade of red as he answered that my Sunday school class had given it to him the night before to give to me, but he had forgotten to bring it into the house. I told him to leave it and we would take it in later since we had already locked up the house.

When we returned home later, he carefully carried the beautiful rose bush into the house. I watered it and placed it on our sun porch so it could revive itself from the overnight stay in the car.

Our son, his wife, and two of their children had come to be with us during the surgery and hospital stay. We spent a great evening talking, but since we had to be up and at the hospital early we decided we had better get to bed.

The next morning I awoke early as usual. It was always around 5:00 a.m., a time that I looked forward to since I could spend it in prayer and Bible study. It was always so quiet with nothing but birds singing to celebrate the arrival of spring. I went into our small den and sat down on the sofa with the Bible in my lap. I always prayed first and asked God to lead me to the Scripture He had for me that day. I began to think of so many Scriptures I had read during this time that were giving me comfort. My mind immediately turned to thoughts of streams in the desert and flowers. I opened my Bible to find Isaiah 35 and, there before me, were verses 1 and 2: "...And the desert shall rejoice and blossom as the rose; It shall blossom abundantly and rejoice, even with joy and singing" (NKJV).

I felt that God had just given me a special message of healing and rejoicing through that passage. I continued in my reading of that chapter, feeling even more that it was meant for me that morning, to give me strength and peace.

Soon everyone was up and getting ready to leave for the hospital. Our daughter and her husband had arrived earlier in the morning. I was at peace with all except one thing. It was concern for my family and friends because we had been told the surgery could be several hours, which it would be. We arrived at the hospital and I checked in, but had time to spend with my family. Some friends had also come to be with us. We gathered together and had a prayer before I was called back to the prep room. Everyone was trying to keep me in good spirits, but I realized that I needed to go to the restroom before they called me back. I excused myself and off to the restroom I went. In a few minutes I returned to the waiting room with all eyes watching me. My name had been called just as I had entered the restroom, but I had not heard it. My husband was on pins and needles. He came up and said they were ready for me. I proudly made my way toward the desk. I wondered why everyone kept watching me when my husband looked back and then quietly whispered into my ear that I had picked up a very long length of toilet tissue going down the side of my slacks. I looked back and it seemed to be flowing for several yards. I reached around and tore it from me with a big laugh. It was very embarrassing but sure provided a bit of humor to everyone! I then gave and received hugs from family and friends and was escorted to the prep room to get the infamous IV, etc. I was sitting up on the bed when a nurse (angel?) came in and told me that a person named Rose would be helping me today. She then left so quickly that I didn't get a chance to question her about it. Did I really hear her correctly? Yes, I did.

Soon three ministers that my husband worked with came to see me. We talked for a while and they had prayer with me. I repeated the story of the rose from the beginning to just what had happened a few minutes ago. They were amazed and rejoiced in how God works in such mysterious ways and in circumstances we can never imagine. The pastors left and then my family members began coming in to pray again and reaffirm to me their support and love. The nurse came in and told them it was about time for me to be taken down to the surgery area. I was left alone for a few minutes and found myself reflecting upon things I had talked with God about over these past few days. One of my major conversations with Him concerned witnessing.

CHAPTER 6: *Be a Witness*

I think most of us as Christians try to be a positive witness for Christ wherever we are. The thought had gone through my mind several times about my life as a Christian witness. This may come as a surprise to some, but I realized that I had let many opportunities to speak God's message to others just go by me. I thought, *It's not the right place* or *It's not the right time.* On and on I could go with excuses! Before the surgery, I prayed and received constant affirmation from God. He was ahead of me in my thoughts and questions. What if I died during surgery? Would God be pleased with my life, my ministry here? Over and over I searched my soul for answers. Finally I received peace from His word, from others, and by His presence in my life.

After doing a review of my life, I realized that witnessing was one area that I definitely was lacking in fulfilling the great commission.

Matthew 28:19–20 says, "Go therefore and make disciples of all the nations, baptizing them in the name of the Father and of the Son and of the Holy Spirit, teaching them to observe all things that I have commanded you; and lo, I am with you always, even to the end of the age." Amen. (NKJV).

Most people would think that I had witnessing down to an art because my husband and I had served as missionaries with the International Mission Board (IMB), the North American Mission Board (NAMB), and Southern Baptist Conservatives of Virginia (SBCV), which are organizations of the Southern Baptist Convention, and had served in several churches in various states. So it hit home with me and I asked God to give me more courage and opportunities to witness. I would take the steps and follow through with my promise to honor Him by sharing His word. At this time, I could not know just what a testimony He was going to give me as a witness for His glory.

I began my new assignment from Him: to witness by praying with my doctors. I had asked God to please let me share with the doctors and team that I am a believer, a Christian, and I wanted them to know that God is the great physician. His son, Jesus, and the Holy Spirit would be in the operating room with them to guide them. All they had to do was to ask on my behalf, even if they were not believers. Oh, the hesitation wanted to creep back in, but I was going to keep my promise to God. Now the time had come to follow through and it began.

I was taken down to the holding area for surgery and soon the anesthesiologist came to talk with me and I asked if I could pray for him. He said he would like that and he reached for my hand. I prayed with him. Soon another person came and again I prayed. Several more doctors came. We held hands and I prayed with them. Yes there were believers there. It had been one of the most precious moments of my life yet. I told the main two who would do the surgery that, no matter what happened in the operating room, I would be okay, and I wanted them to be okay with whatever, if anything happened to me. They assured me they were going to do their best and believed all would be just fine. During all this *witnessing,* the whole area was so quiet you could hear the proverbial pin drop.

My husband and I were left alone for a few minutes and I told him that I felt that I was surrounded by "something." He said he could feel it also. I don't know if it was angels or the Holy Spirit, but definitely God had a hold on me.

Shortly thereafter a man came and I was on my way to the operating room. We traveled down a long hallway and I began talking to the man escorting me. I asked if he was a Christian—a believer. He answered with a strong response, "Yes, ma'am." I again asked if he had ever accepted Christ as his personal Savior. Before he could answer, another person appeared in the hallway and said something to the effect of "If you don't have the Man, you don't have anything. If you got the Man, you got everything," and that person began praising the Lord. My escort laughed and said that he was a Sunday school teacher and he had accepted Christ as his Savior a long time ago. There were amens in the hallway and I could feel the very strong presence of the Holy Spirit.

Be careful what you pray for. God didn't wait long to bring my request for witnessing before me. It was not Samaria, Judea, or a foreign field, but right here in Virginia in a hospital bed on my way to surgery for stage-three thyroid cancer.

I had kept my promise to God and knew that if I came out of surgery without a voice that I would use sign language or whatever to be a faithful witness for Him. Little did I know what He was preparing for me and what He would use for me to be His witness. I again recalled the Scripture that I had read earlier in Isaiah 35:1–2: "As a rose blooms in the desert …" (NKJV). Little did I know just what this Scripture would come to mean to me every day since. I thought about the rose bush and how people will just pass by a rose bush that has not bloomed. When a rose bush has tiny buds, they will stop and give it a quick glance. They will wonder just what kind of rose it will be, what its color will be. But if you take a rose bush that is almost in full bloom, people will stop, look, touch, and even grab a quick sniff. They stand back and admire it and then go on their way with a pleasant smile and the sweet aroma of the rose. It has had an effect on their life. That was what I wanted my life to be: like a rose, to have an effect on the soul of others, to bloom for God, to be as the rose in the desert to make a difference in the lives of others. My journey continues.

CHAPTER 7: *Into Surgery*

I was wheeled into the surgery room and went through the usual process of being transferred to the operating bed. I remembered praying and feeling a great sense of peace as I entered the cold room. I was still excited about having the opportunity to witness and pray with some of the people around me. I knew God had everything in His control and no matter what happened I would be just fine. I had accepted that so many things could always go wrong and the biggest concern was just how much of the growth was attached to the vocal chords, if any. Now as I was ready to be put into la-la land, as we often refer to being put to sleep, I gave everything to God and knew He would give me strength to handle whatever the outcome would be. I had claimed healing and I was holding fast to that.

The next thing I knew was feeling a horrible pain in my neck. I could hear the doctors speaking and words such as, "it's bad, it's really bad." I could hear their conversation and I wanted so desperately to be able to speak and tell them to please be quiet. Didn't they know that I could hear their every word? *Please don't say those things while I am lying here totally helpless.* How could they know just how bad the cancer was? Then the pain overtook their conversation. I silently cried out to God. *Please God, take away this horrible pain, pain that I had never experienced before.* I knew I was lying down and it was impossible for me to get up or talk. I felt that I had reached the brink of death and called out in a silent voice for God. I then felt my body begin to rise up. I thought, *I know that I am ready to be with you, God. I am ready to leave this earth, but please be with my family as they sit in the waiting room. Give them peace, God, the peace I have now.*

Suddenly I found myself in the waiting room observing my family and friends. A door opened and I saw the doctor come in. My husband came up immediately to him, followed by my son and daughter. They were smiling and feeling that things had gone so well with the surgery, but their smiles were soon gone as the doctor told them that something had gone wrong. I did not make it through surgery. I immediately saw the look on my husband's face. I felt as if I was him and I could feel every emotion he had. It was such a feeling of desolation, abandonment, and total despair. I felt emotions he had for me that I did not think were possible on earth. I wanted to cry out to him, but I could not because at that moment I was within him, feeling his every emotion. Then I was *transferred*, for lack of a better word, into my son. I felt his sudden feeling as if he was a small child left alone in a dark, vast desert and he had a complete emptiness as if all his blood had drained out of his body and into the floor. It was as if he looked down and could see his blood pooled around him, yet he kept standing there with such emptiness and numbness.

I again was *transferred* to my daughter to feel her emotion. Hers was one of shock and disbelief. How could this happen, how does one survive without her mother? She too felt the desolation and the emptiness of loss. She felt her body turn cold but struggled to find words to reassure her dad and brother. She felt a maternal instinct unlike any she had ever felt. This was all strange and unreal.

I felt the sadness, shock, and humbleness the doctor felt as he walked to my family. As I began to see the scene before me and all the tears I could not cry, the arms that could not embrace them, and the words I could not speak, I cannot find words to this day to describe how much I loved them.

Suddenly I heard a soft wonderful sound. It was music so unlike any I had ever heard. It gave me peace and led me to forget and turn from my family. I wanted to stay with them, but the music was so overpowering to my soul that I had to follow the sound. I was immediately back in the operating room and once again lying on my surgical bed. I knew I could not turn my head, but my eyes were able to turn toward the music. My eyes then saw off to the right what seemed to be a soft but glowing light surrounding people. My first thought was, *Why are all these people standing there watching me?* I then became aware that they didn't seem to be people, but yet they were. They radiated such peace, light, gentleness, and love that it gave me peace. Suddenly I realized there were only four people. They were all dressed alike in white robes and each had identical golden hair unlike the golden hair we have on earth. I watched as they were looking at me and very quickly I saw them, in unison, turn their heads to their right in perfect precision. They looked up to their right at the exact moment a different music sounded again. This music had a force to it, something that made me realize something or someone very important was coming. I was reminded of "Hail to the Chief," the song that is played when the president of the United States is about to make a formal appearance. Of course, the *presidential* music could never compare to this music. It just about took my breath away! It was so totally commanding and beautiful. There are no words to express these sounds of music.

Again the music changed, this time into a much softer and more comforting sound as my eyes turned to my left. I began to feel that I was being lifted up, but I knew that I had to still be lying on the bed. Or was I? I followed the music as I began to see a white mist. It was like a heavy fog yet was not wet. I felt it was somewhat like a beautiful snow with extremely small round snow pellets falling before me but not touching me. I watched as the mist gradually disappeared into a mixture of magnificent lights, a magnificent rainbow of glorious colors. It encompassed me into a peacefulness and beauty unlike anything I had ever seen or felt. I am still unable to describe everything I saw.

The music changed to a different sound and I saw billows of white fluffy something. I followed the billows until I realized it was a long white robe. The robe had something within its folds that held my attention until it reached the shoulder of the robe. I saw long white hair that matched the robe, but I could not see who it was. The light, a brilliant golden color, was so bright that I could not keep my eyes focused. It reminded me of the sun at day and the moon at night shining together as one. I was caught up in the beauty and tranquility of everything when I heard someone laugh and call my name, "Linda, I am here," He said. Everything else stopped. The beauty of it all and the sound of the voice made me feel that nothing else existed, that time was standing still. Nothing else existed and again words and description escape me.

I don't know how long I was in this place, but at some point I realized I must be lying on a bed again. He stepped out of this place that I have seen and took two more steps. I knew then that He was coming to me. I cried out to Him that He could not come to me. He is Holy. His love encompassed me and I felt Him so near that the sleeve of His robe touched my left arm. I still get chills on my arm after these two and one-half years when I remember the touch of that robe. Many times I will find myself remembering what I experienced, so much so, that my eyes fill to overflowing with tears of amazement and love for my Lord. I have no explanation for what happened to me.

I know that God has different ways He may reveal Himself to us. I don't spend time trying to explain what happened to me or why it happened. Did I really wake up in surgery? Did God take this opportunity to reveal Himself to me in this special way? I do know that my life has been changed. I know that I have been able to comfort people who are dying. I tell them that heaven is so awesome. Our God is there to receive us if we have repented of our sins and accepted Christ as our Savior and Lord. I just tell myself that God has surely given me an answer to my prayer in helping me be a witness for Him. Be careful what you ask for.

Sometime later, I became aware that I was hearing the voices of my family. I slowly opened my eyes and there stood my husband, daughter, and son. They told me the surgery had gone well but was long. I signed that Jesus loved me. I was so very happy. My husband wanted to lead in a prayer of thanksgiving for God being so good to us. My son then spoke up and looked at me and told me that he just knew that I could talk. Where his words came from I didn't know. I had already been told that my voice might take a while to come back and then we still would not know if there would be permanent damage. Did he know something the rest of us didn't know? I then opened my mouth and spoke the words that I wanted to lead the prayer. Much to our surprise, I was able to be heard as I prayed. Here I was just coming out of several hours of surgery in the neck area and now I was voicing a prayer to God!

I would yet have a long journey to complete healing of the voice, but God had just shown us that He had begun the healing process. God is so great.

CHAPTER 8: God's Continuous Work

God has continued to work in my life to give me peace and reaffirm His healing of my body. I had been recovering and I knew others were still praying for me. I could feel their love and support as I went through the days after surgery, but now it was time for my check-up.

I had gotten up early as usual and had my prayer and Bible study. I must admit that I had a few moments of *what-ifs*. I guess that comes to all who have been faced with serious situations and health issues. I always felt God letting me know He was with me. The Holy Spirit was the one here on earth that gave me the comfort and would guide me through each phase of my recovery. I grew to depend on Him constantly.

The day for my check-up came and I felt a peace knowing I would hear from the doctors themselves just how the surgery had gone. I wondered if they really knew what had gone on in the operating room. I decided to wait and see how they felt about the surgery and what my prognosis would be.

It was time now for my husband and me to make our trip to the doctor's office, and I felt another kind of emotion. Did I really wake up during surgery? Did anything happen during surgery that we were not told about? I knew that this had really happened to me, but I had not shared it with anyone until the night before my check-up.

My husband and I were sitting on the front porch of our house. He was in his white wicker rocking chair and I was in mine. He pointed out to me that I had been unusually quiet today and wanted to know if I was worried about the upcoming check-up. I told him no, that I was not really worried about the check-up, but it was something else that had happened to me during surgery. I hesitated to share it with him.

Well, never make that statement to your husband or you will peak his curiosity and he will never let you rest until you tell him. I told him the events of everything that I had experienced during surgery and that I wanted God to confirm it. He looked at me the whole time I was talking. I wondered if he would think I was crazy or what. I finally finished the story, except the part of the doctor coming out to say that I had not made it through surgery. I did not think at the time to share all that, so I just shared the part with the angels and God.

He commented on all the "scenes," as he called them, and said we could ask the doctor tomorrow. I prayed for God to give me the words to say and when to say them to the doctors. Now I had to wait for tomorrow.

The next morning, as we continued our trip to the doctor's office, I again reminded my husband about the experience. When we arrived, we were shown into his office without much wait time. My stomach was churning, but still I knew that I had been in the presence of God Almighty no matter what the doctor would say. I felt I would not need anyone's assurance of what had happened, but I would ask anyway. After the exam, while both doctors were in the room, I asked, "Which one of you said …?" and I quoted the words. Suddenly one doctor sat down on the desk and said that I had to be awake during that time to have heard what I did. The other doctor said, "I said those words when I examined you before." I said, "No, you never said these words to me." They suddenly became very quiet. I knew they were great doctors and I would never hesitate to use them again or recommend them to anyone. They could not have known what I was going through because God had blocked my pain after a few sentences from them. God was showing me He was dealing with *me,* not them.

CHAPTER 9: *Finger Paints*

Shortly after my surgery, I was lying on my sofa trying to get a nap before starting dinner. My husband had made it very clear that I was to get a nap every afternoon, and he did not want to hear any excuses of why I should not take a nap. This was always hard for me since I have always been an active person. Going through this cancer had just presented a challenge for me to stay active. Nevertheless I decided I would try to be an obedient wife and take the nap or just rest if I could not sleep. I had been lying there on that old leather sofa all covered with my favorite burgundy blanket when I decided that I had had enough of this. I thought I could read some in the Bible or just talk to God, but instead I found myself reflecting on the surgery and the events that had transpired. I became concerned that I had not written everything down about the *visitation*. I began asking God to *please never, never let that event leave my mind.* I said to Him to please let that memory remain with me throughout my life. It was such a special life-changing event for me.

Suddenly I heard a voice saying that I should paint it. *Paint what?* I said in my mind.

Paint the picture, the voice repeated.

I answered with a *Well, just how can I paint that picture? I hate to color, always have, and don't intend to start now. Painting, I can't paint.* I laughed and thought that perhaps I was dreaming or having a nightmare really. *Painting, are you crazy?* I said again to myself.

I lay back down on the sofa, but I became more restless with these thoughts going through my mind: *paint and you won't forget*. I repeated again, *I can't paint.*

The question came back to me. *You have fingers, don't you?*

Fingers, *yes, I have fingers.*

Well, use the fingers to paint with.

Back and forth my argument went until I said in a defeated tone, *okay, I will finger-paint*. By this time, my husband was home from work so we ate dinner, watched TV, and I soon forgot about the finger-painting episode.

The next morning, as I was eating my breakfast of hot oatmeal and drinking my hot tea with milk, I was reminded of the painting conversation the evening before. I began making excuses as to why I definitely could not paint a picture. I could not find one that would get me off the hook about painting. I cleaned up the breakfast dishes, showered, and dressed to go to the mall. I began thinking to myself, *where can I find finger paints and what kind of paper will I use?* Finally, I had come to the fork of the road, so to speak, and made a decision, thanks to a red light stopping me. I decided to head to an art store. I spent time looking but felt that things were too expensive. I could not find what I wanted. This was just another excuse, because the store really had everything anyone could want in paints and papers.

I finally left and thought about going back home, but no there was a Super Store so, to be honest with myself, I thought I had better check it out. I drove over to the store, got out, and went in thinking just how stupid I felt. Perhaps if I had small children I could justify buying finger paints. I couldn't find the paints, so I decided I had better ask a salesclerk to clear my conscience when I arrived home without anything. Wouldn't you know it? Right then a clerk came up to me and asked if I needed help. Perhaps she heard me talking to myself and thought I had lost my mind or something worse. I told her what I was looking for and she remarked something about my children using the paints in school. She was walking toward the hobby area and pointing to the array of paints, brushes, and art boards. She told me the paints were not toxic and would be safe for my children. I wanted to tell her my children were too old to finger-paint, but I knew I had to be nice and appreciate the compliment whether she meant it or not. I wanted to get away from her and get on my way, but she asked what type and size board I would need or did the children just use something called "butcher paper" or whatever.

I finally pulled myself together and thought, *Just how is she going to feel when I admit that all these painting supplies are for me?* When I told her they were not for children but for me, she looked a bit embarrassed. I had no choice but to tell her my experience in the operating room and what I wanted to do. She was very quiet and, when I finished, she continued to look at me and then she spoke. I could not believe it, but she was really touched. She remarked how wonderful it was that God revealed Himself to me and what He had done and was doing with me. Needless to say, I was humbled that it took a Super Store clerk to help me see that God was still using me, and, even if I could not paint, I had to be obedient to Him. I thanked her and turned to walk to the check-out to pay for my painting supplies. I began looking around the store and wondering just how many of the people I saw were Christians. How many were lost and would never choose to experience salvation or the beauty of God and His love for them? I said a silent prayer for them, paid for my supplies, and walked out to the car with a new attitude. God was already using me as a witness to His wonderful plan.

I arrived home, went to my kitchen, and spread out all the paints and the white poster board on the table. I said a prayer of commitment to God to do my best to be obedient in what He wanted me to do. I began.

I remembered what the clerk had said about nontoxic paints, so I stuck my fingers in the jar of white paint and put them upon the white board. Okay! White on white! "Wasn't that real smart?" I said to myself. But if I had purchased any other color, nothing else would have turned out right. The painting wasn't going to any art gallery or to win a prize, so I continued to paint. I put the angels where I remembered they stood, the rainbow, everything I could remember. I came to the hands of the angels but had no way to do them until I spied a tiny mascara brush on the windowsill. I thought that would be perfect for making fingers.

Soon the picture was as complete as I could get it. I was glad I had finished it because my husband had decided to come home early from work. He was in the kitchen looking over my shoulder. He looked at me like, *yes, you have finally lost your mind.* I believe he was ready to call the doctor. I told him not to worry, but I was just being obedient. Well, that was a new one for him because I do have a bit of a "stubborn streak," as he calls it. I then began to explain to him just what I painted. He started laughing and telling me that I basically had wasted my time because the colors would not show up on the white board. White on white would definitely not work. He told me that after dinner we would go out and get a different color and a better board for me to use. I told him that I appreciated his interest, but this was the way it would remain. No rerun on the painting. I took the painting off the kitchen counter and laid it on the dining room table in the other room. "Now," I said to myself, "I am through with that!" I gathered up the paints, put them into their box, and set them in a cabinet. *I am glad that is over,* I thought. Little did I know what was in store for that picture.

The next morning we got up and I went into the dining room to see if the picture was dry. I wanted to store it in the closet just as a reminder of what had happened to me. I knew it was not to be artwork on any wall in my house. I saw that it was dry and picked it up to take to the closet in another room when my husband said he wanted to see it. I put it back on the table and, much to my surprise he remarked how unusual it was. *Okay,* I thought, you don't have to insult me. But then I looked at the picture and I could not believe it. There were folds painted into the robe and, yes, you could see white on white, but with definition. So much had changed in the picture, things that I had not put in it. We both knew that only God could have done that. The picture is not a *masterpiece* in man's terminology, but in our minds it is a special blessing from God. Yes, it would never get a prize or find a place in anyone else's home, but it has a treasured place in our hearts and home. We love it and thank God for showing us in that special way that He can take our obedience to Him and give us an unexpected blessing.

CHAPTER 10: *Radioactive Treatment*

Shortly after my cancer surgery, I was scheduled for a full body scan. Since I am not in the medical field, I will not discuss the medical part of this treatment. I will share with you some of the things I could and could not do after taking a radioactive pill which was necessary for the scan.

My husband and I met with the doctor and he explained why he recommended this scan and the precautions we would need to take once I swallowed the pill. I would have to be on a special no-iodine diet. I do not mind saying that was a difficult diet at first. I had never realized just how many foods contained iodine or iodized salt. I received a list of some of the "forbidden" foods, which helped with the diet. The food I ate could contain the non-iodized salt but, for the most part, I just left salt out of my food. This diet would last for a short while. The fun part of this diet, or at least for a couple of days, was that my husband had to do all the cooking. Since I was somewhat radioactive, I could not use the kitchen because I would leave the area "contaminated." My husband was so proud of himself, going to the grocery store, planning the menu, and cooking. I had delicious meals, such as cooked oatmeal for breakfast with black coffee or tea and sometimes fresh fruit. Lunch and dinner he toiled over for seemingly hours before he brought the array of somewhat overcooked food to the bedroom.

"Bedroom," did I say? Yes, it was the bedroom. I again would "contaminate" any area where I went, so I chose to stay in the master bedroom. That of course meant that since he could not sit with me to eat, he would have to bring a chair outside the bedroom door and hold his plate on his lap. "We could at least be somewhat together," he said. Then he would give me a breakdown of what was happening at church and outside the house. I think he talked so much just to distract me from asking about the condition of the kitchen. After we ate, I would have to throw my paper plate, plastic silverware, and cup in a small garbage bag. He would gather it up carefully, wearing rubber gloves, and take it out. At first, the meals went great, but in a few days my appetite was totally lost. He purchased fresh fruit, sodas, dessert, whatever he could find to whet my appetite, but the food had begun to taste the same. Only through his encouragement and pushing me did I eat. He really was so great during his chef days.

I mentioned that I occupied the master bedroom and, yes, I did. We were told we had to stay several feet apart and that meant in the bedroom, kitchen, car, and wherever we were. It was total isolation to him. I did give him his favorite pillow and told him he could enjoy his snoring since he would be in another bedroom.

I could not go out in public because of contamination. I learned that one could only watch so much television or read so many books. I have never been one to be bored, but now I had learned what people, and especially my children, meant when they said they were bored.

It was amazing how much God taught me during that time of somewhat isolation. I put myself in the place of people in nursing homes, the critically ill, disabled, and homebound people. I never knew I would miss my church family and services as I did. I spent time on the phone, but it was definitely not the same as face-to-face fellowship.

Finally the day came that I could be out in the world again. Oh, to see my kitchen, even if I had to completely rearrange things in the cabinets and clean the refrigerator and stove! My husband and I agreed that cooking and cleaning were not his gifts, and I certainly did not have the gift of patience. It had taken cancer to show us many things about ourselves.

We would learn more about each other and ourselves when we went into the doctor's office to get the report of the test after taking the radioactive pill. This was a bit scary to face the doctor again. We had claimed healing and we were very much at peace believing all was well. I know that no matter how much faith one has, Satan likes to cause us to doubt. I do admit that when those thoughts came into my mind, I reminded myself of what had happened to me in the operating room. I knew God had complete control over my life. I knew that any type of doubt was not what I would accept for myself. Now I faced the doctor for the follow-up results.

We sat and listened to the doctor and saw the report. We gave God the praise that all was well. God had done wonderful and marvelous things for us. The cancer had attached itself to a part of my body that could have resulted in loss of voice. God had provided excellent doctors and medical staff to take the cancer from me. God had used the doctors, medical staff, and prayers of many people for my healing. My voice was preserved to be used to praise Him aloud for what He had done for me.

My husband and I left the doctor's office with a skip in our steps, thanksgiving in our hearts, and vocal praise to Him. Oh, by the way, we stopped for a nice yummy meal on the way home. Amen.

CHAPTER 11: *Moving On*

The weeks and months began going by quickly. I kept my check-up appointments with the doctors and each time I received good reports. Everything was going well to a quick recovery. My voice had been affected somewhat, but it was not long before I was sharing my testimony at church and other places. During all the recovery, we also sold our home and moved closer to our church. The long drive to and from church was taking its toll on us. We found a beautiful townhome and were rejoicing in the goodness of our Lord when things began to change. My husband accepted a staff position with a church in another part of the state. Here I was facing another move.

I questioned if God was really calling us to another church so soon. I had just had major surgery the last of April, sold a home, packed, and moved to another home in September and now a few months later He was asking us to move again. Never argue with God, because you will lose the argument. I complained, but it didn't do any good. I said that I wasn't able to make such a drastic change so soon after surgery. It didn't help. I knew it was time to accept the call to another location, another church, and, most of all, the change of such great doctors. I loved my church, the pastor, and the people. I loved and enjoyed the area of the state we lived in and I didn't understand why we should move. Why move when things are going so well?

The Holy Spirit sure got a workout when the time came to leave our townhome, church, and family. In March, eleven months after surgery for stage-three thyroid cancer, I was facing a new church and church family, another home to get in order again, a new location, and, with a bit of panic, new doctors. To make things worse, I was facing my yearly check-up and I truly needed to rely on God. I was mentally and physically exhausted by the end of our move at the end of March.

God was right there providing us with a beautiful home to live in and another great church and church family. I still had to find the doctor for my yearly check-up. God sent us some friends to refer us to a doctor who was able to see me quickly. Getting medical records and scheduling the body scan were not as easy as we had expected, but, after some time, we were able to get the body scan done. Praise the Lord. All went well and there was no sign of the cancer. I know that it would have been impossible for me to survive that first year had it not been God giving me abundant strength. He also gave us two great churches filled with a great support of prayers and love.

The time passed quickly and I had my two year check-up in June. This time it was not a full body scan but a scan of the neck area. This would be an easier scan. I would not have to take the radioactive pill or be on a special diet. I would not have to give my kitchen over to my husband again. We were most thankful for that. Give him Italian spaghetti to cook and he is great. Perhaps because he is Italian, he thinks everything should have tomatoes in it. Anyway, we knew this scan would be so much easier and less stressful, or so we thought.

I went into the hospital outpatient area and the scan began. After several minutes, the tech doing the scan told me she had to go into the other room to have the scan checked. That is the normal procedure. Sometime later she came back in and told me that the radiologist would be checking the scan, but she had to do another scan first. Another scan was done and again she went out, and several minutes later she came in again and told me the radiologist may want to come in and do another scan. She left the room and I realized that something had to be wrong. The scan must have shown something because I didn't think the radiologist would do the scan if things were okay

I lay back onto the bed and began to pray. I reminded God that I had claimed healing and I was still holding on to it. I realized that Satan was trying to get me scared, to doubt, and to control my innermost thoughts. I said to God that I knew He was in control of my life and I would not give Satan that control. I could feel the tumult of the air in the room and I spoke out loudly to Satan. I told him that I would not accept his trying to control me. I told him that he would need to go to God, not me, because I was God's creation and I belonged to Him. I felt the air clear and had peace and comfort.

Suddenly the door to the room opened and in walked the tech and the radiologist. The radiologist said the tech had found an area she was concerned about and he wanted to check it himself. Well, I knew then that God had already taken care of everything and there would be nothing there that should not be. The test began again and for several minutes there was only the sound of the machine. The radiologist spoke quietly and asked the tech if the area he was checking was what she had seen and was questioning. She said, "Yes, that was the spot." He continued his checking of the area and told me that she had questioned the spot, and then, after a few minutes, he told her that nothing unusual was there. It was nothing. I was giving God thanks silently when the radiologist asked her if she had checked the other area of the neck. Her reply was "No." He asked me what type of cancer I had and asked a few more questions. He then told her that in this type of cancer, the other side of the neck area had to be checked because the cancer could sometimes spread there. I took it as another attempt by Satan to make me fall apart. He had tried so much that day to get me upset. I continued to lay still and pray. The doctor finished the test and walked away to wash his hands, then turned around and told me that everything looked fine. He said he could not see any signs of the cancer but I should keep my appointments with my doctor. I told him that I had been praying and I appreciated him and thanked him.

I dressed and the tech and I walked back to the waiting room to get my husband. On the way, I again questioned her and she said everything was fine. We began talking and I told her of my belief and she shared that she was a Christian and believed in healing too. *Isn't our God great?*

It has been two and one-half years since the surgery, and God has done so very much for me and my family. I have shared my testimony with many, many others and have had opportunities that I could never have had if I had not had cancer. God has performed so many miracles in my life and used me in ways that I could never have imagined.

CHAPTER 12: *No Journey Back*

In the beginning of the book I wrote about "no journey back." I have and continue to be on a journey that I did not plan or desire to take. In truth, when first diagnosed with cancer, I had the thought flash across my mind that my life could end quickly, but God has been my gracious, loving, and a steadfast companion. He was on this journey preparing the way before I even took my first step with cancer.

I am a different person today and I thank God for all He has done and is doing for and with me. Witnessing and giving encouragement, I have shared my testimony with many people. I often make a statement that surprises them, both Christian and non-Christian. I tell them that if God told me I could go back and skip the cancer but I would remain the same person, I would not want that life again. I would rather have had cancer if that was the only way I could experience God, growth, and a more meaningful life with Him. God has taught me more in these couple of years than over the many years of my lifetime.

I did find one area of frustration with my feelings a few weeks after surgery. I would think about the rainbow and its colors, but I could never find colors here that looked the same. I realized most of the colors I had seen throughout my *surgery* experience did not look the same here. Then I felt as if something from my life was missing; a part of me was gone. I finally talked to my husband about it and he laughed and said that it was the cancer that was missing. I finally told him that I felt like I had left a part of me in heaven. How can I explain that? I had experienced such beauty, peace, and, well, I still cannot explain it all.

The music was another area that I missed hearing. Sometimes I would walk through the house and suddenly hear the sounds in my mind, but it was still not the same. I finally began to concentrate on the things I had to do to get back into the *full swing of things* here. Little did I know what else God had in store for me.

A few months ago, I began having the sounds of music come back very strongly in my life. I would tell God that I sure wished He had given me the gift of a great singer or, better yet, the gift of being a great pianist. Perhaps I could satisfy my soul through my own musical ability. I would then laugh and think, *What a joke that is to think I could ever have any musical abilities.*

Yet God surprised me in a way that was so unexpected. One night, as I went upstairs to bed, I heard a song—words and music—in my head. I lay down in bed and tried to go to sleep, but I heard, "Get up and write the words down." I was trying to be obedient, so I went into the office beside the bedroom and picked up a pencil and paper. I walked into the hall bathroom and, by the light of a tiny nightlight, I wrote the words down. It took me about two minutes because the words were coming so fast. I walked back into the bedroom and my husband asked if I was okay. I told him I was fine but I wanted to read him some words I had written for a song. He was so quiet that I thought he had gone to sleep. He asked about the music for the song and I told him that he was to play notes on the keyboard and I would tell him the "sounds" to use for the song. Believe it or not, he did not laugh, but he looked at me strangely. The next morning we began the hunt-and-peck system for the music. He has been so great in getting the song and music written and we both think it is good. Yes, he agreed, it was a strange way to put a song together, but it worked.

A week or so later, my husband and I were working in our home office—he on something for church and I on family history. I had gotten up from my desk to go downstairs to get us a snack when I heard the music again. This time was different because I could hear a song—words and music together—along with seeing a video playing in my mind. I stopped when I heard the words for me to write it all down. I took a piece of paper and pencil from the desk and began writing the words along with a description of what the video should be. I turned to my husband and handed him the paper. He looked at me and rolled his eyes. He asked if the music was going to be chosen the same way as for the other song. I told him, "Yes, it would be the hunt-and-peck system again." The song is nearing completion, and we hope to begin our work on the video in the coming weeks. I just pray it will all be done for God's glory. As Phillip was playing the song a couple of days ago, he mentioned that it had such a "spiritual" message.

The following event happened first, but I wanted to save it for last since it is the most unbelievable for both of us. It was about two months or so before the above songs were written. I had finished my prayer and Bible study time and leaned back on the sofa to close my eyes for a few minutes. I think this was the first time in a while that I heard music again. I thought that if I were gifted in music, I could go sit and play the keyboard. I knew that was impossible, but I heard the words to write the notes down. Musical notes like A, B, and C, they were mixed up to me and I had no idea what I had to write down, but I wrote down everything I was told. I felt like an idiot. I put the paper in my Bible and leaned back on the sofa again. I was told to tell my husband that he was to play this "music." Well, my thoughts were that he would definitely laugh me out of the house. Then I heard, "I will prove to him that he is to do this." I picked up the paper and wrote the notes as I was told.

It was a late day for my husband at church and I was so excited, but hesitant, for him to get home. Finally he arrived home and, after he had rested for a while, I told him I had something I wanted him to play. "Notes on the keyboard," I told him. I wanted to hear what they sounded like. I gave him the paper and he began to play. I was so nervous and scared because he didn't say anything. Then I heard the words to tell him to change and do this and that with the notes. I was totally at a loss on what I was saying. I didn't understand anything, but I told him what I had been told. He looked at me and asked where I got the notes. I asked him if it was really bad and he replied that they were fine, but he wanted to know where I got them. He even had the nerve to ask if I had gotten them from a television show or computer. I told him, "No, I got them from God." He laughed and asked where I had really gotten them. I then was told to tell him to add something different to the notes. I immediately told him what I had just been told and he turned and began playing. I had no idea if any of this made sense, because it was something he would never have thought about playing. He really shocked me when he remarked that, even with his doctorate in music from a well-known university, he found the music unique and unusual.

He is now working on this composition. I am amazed that God has chosen this time in my husband's life and my life to put us together for this music. Why has God done this for me especially? I don't know, but I have learned to be more open to His words and work in my life. I just cannot imagine what my life would have been like if I had not had cancer. I would have missed out on so many wonderful blessings. He was there before the journey and still walks the journey with me. *No journey back, no journey back.* There is so much to look forward to when the journey is over.

A little blonde, skinny-legged girl running down the road in a small coal-mining town. A scared little girl yelling to the chosen men, "Come quick, Charlie needs you!" A little girl standing in the shadow of her grandmother watching and listening to men pray. A little girl filled with thanks and wonder that such a simple thing as prayer made her beloved grandfather get out of bed, walk, drink coffee from a saucer, and hold her again.

A glowing bride filled with joy and happiness in knowing this is the plan and person God has chosen for her.

A student wife working to help support her husband as he finishes college and enters seminary. A wife who will learn how to proofread a thesis at midnight because her husband is studying for the upcoming exams.

A young wife who now becomes a mother. A dear, sweet, precious baby who comes a few days before Christmas. One who now made us a true family. Three years later, another blessing for a precious son to be born to enrich the family.

A maturing woman. One who has survived months of colicky babies, cuts, and bruises on growing toddlers and tears shed as they leave for their first day of school. Not so many tears when they leave for high school, but lots of tears when they take off for college.

A more mature woman. It's her grandchildren whom she rocked when they had colic. The wonderful grandchildren to bless her life. To see and hear about their lives and her prayers for their future.

A blessed woman, mother, grandmother. A woman who still sees the God she learned to love and accept as a child, the God who never changes. A God that has and is changing her. A woman who has survived crying, colicky babies, teenagers, marriage, many *church* moves, cancer, and sometime in the future a stay-at-home husband.

God has been her constant companion and her constant help. She could not have completed the journey this far without Him and His many blessings. He is faithful, *always*. Her greatest journey is still ahead.

A skinny-legged young girl running with her long blonde pigtails flying in the air, a grandmother with short blonde hair being ruffled by the gentle breeze. The young girl *saw* healing taking place but the grandmother *has* and is still *experiencing* healing. The same healer of years ago is still the same healer of today and all the tomorrows.

The *journey* continues. *No journey back! No journey back!*

The beginning direction for your journey can be found in the Bible at John 3:16–17: "For God so loved the world that He gave His only begotten Son, that whoever believes in Him should not perish but have everlasting life. For God did not send His Son into the world to condemn the world, but that the world through Him might be saved" (NKJV).

If you want to be a part of this journey, follow these directions for a successful and joyful trip.

Amen and amen.

CHAPTER 13: *Generation to Generation*

In chapter three of this book I wrote about my prayer for healing and my desire to live to see my children grow old and experience the beauty of being grandparents. I wanted to see my grandchildren graduate from high school and college, to attend their weddings and to be there when my great grandchildren are born. I still had lots of things I wanted to do for God and I wanted to live to accomplish them. I quoted the scripture from Isaiah 51:8 about generation to generation and I claimed that verse as my daily scripture of hope.

When the previous chapter, "No Journey Back" was written I thought about other stories I had wanted to include but was unsure as to whether the stories were relevant. I now believe that God knew all along that I should include these stories in this book in order to show the spiritual influences that so many have had on my life. I pray that these stories will enlighten you as to who I am and encourage you to leave a part of your heritage in written form for your future generations.

Throughout the years I have worked on my family's history but for more than just to know about who was who. I wanted to know the kind of people from whom I had descended. I knew that the Bible contained much about the genealogy of Jesus and I wondered how many Godly people existed in my past. Did they leave me a heritage of Godly principles? Would their prayers have been for future generations of grandchildren, *generation to generation*? Did their faith in God help build my faith?

I now know that, yes, they did leave me a Godly heritage; a heritage that I am destined and determined to pass on to the next generation.

Each generation has to make their own decision as to how they will live their lives and what they will leave for their future family heritage. It is my prayer that my generation will leave a Godly heritage for the generation that follows. It was the faith of those in the past that has helped to build my faith. A faith that has sustained me in my battle with cancer.

I have always been interested in the history of all of my family. I knew my paternal grandfather had descended from German linage but I did not know much about my grandmother. My maternal grandfather was said to have descended from a Native American Indian heritage and my grandmother was of Scottish descent. One day I asked my maternal grandmother, Ma, to tell me about her and grandfather's family. She began giving me as much information as she could and more than I could write down at the time. Once she shared an interesting story about what my grandfather did for me when I was born. It was fascinating to me then and continues to be so today. I have written it with all of the details and background told to me by *Ma*.

MESSAGE

My family has left me a Godly heritage. I have recently found one member that served as a pastor of two churches in the 1700's and another born in early 1800's was said to have *"healing powers"*. It was noted that he was a very Godly Man. I know I am blessed to have had many such great men of God in my past. Their message of faith in God has been passed down from generation to generation.

SONG: FAITH OF OUR FATHER'S

CHAPTER 14: *The Blessing*

It was a cold day in the small coal mining town of southwestern Virginia. Snow flurries flew around in the harsh wind that seemed to find its way into every nook and cranny of the small four room house. The two coal burning stoves could not produce enough heat to keep the whole house warm. The kitchen stove kept the kitchen warm and the big "*Warm Morning*" stove in the living/bedroom kept that room warm but did not heat the bedroom where my mother was lying in bed with labor pains. She was living with her parents while my dad was away in the military. I would be mother's first child.

It was about sunset in the evening when mother gave birth to me. She told me later that even though she was worn out from the hours of labor, she was excited about the birth of her baby girl. I had just been cleaned up and put in a warm gown when my grandfather walked in from his work in the coal mine near the house. Ma told him that he was a grandfather again. He quickly went into the bedroom, looked at me for a moment or two, reached over and grabbed a small blanket and gently lifted me up. Once I was wrapped in the blanket, he took me outside onto the cold front porch. He sat down in the old green rocking chair, held me close and whispered in my ear. After some time had passed, he stood up. Ma thought he was bringing me back into the house but to her shock, he loosened the blanket from around me and laid me in his hands. He then lifted me up with his arms fully extended and began saying something which Ma could not understand. She yelled at him to cover me up and get me back into the house before I caught my *death of cold*. He did not acknowledge her but instead pulled me back to his chest and whispered into my ear again. Finally, as she was about to take the broom to his backside, he turned, took me back into the house and placed me beside my mother.

Ma asked him why he had taken me out in weather like that and why had he lifted me up. She had lots of questions for him but he would not tell her anything except it was something his family had done for generations. She told him that he had not done that to any of their children so why did he do that to me. He thought for a moment and told her that it was to pass his children and go to one of his grandchildren and I was the one he passed it on to.

Ma continued to ask him over the years what he had said to me. She wanted to find out more about the *ceremony*. She never received an answer except to say *that Linda will know what I said to her when the time is right and you will know only if she wants to tell you*. Needless to say, Ma continued to ask him and me but neither gave her an answer. Over the years she told me the story many times. It was always the same.

I sometimes thought about the talks Pa and I had when we were alone walking in the woods or working in the garden. I never told her about these but here again she never asked me about them. I remembered that one time when Pa and I were alone that I asked him about a rain dance. He showed me but told me never to tell Ma or she would get mad. Hopefully, one day I can find out if he indeed was of Native Indian heritage.

Years passed and both of these precious grandparents died. I always wondered if Mother could verify the story, *"my blessing"* as I called it. I had never mentioned it to her and realized I would need to ask her soon because she was dying from cancer. The opportunity came while I was visiting with her at the hospital. We had been talking for awhile about many things when she grew tired and we entered into a few minutes of quite time. I felt that this was the moment for me to ask her about the time when I was born.

I had written the story down earlier but had changed the names of everyone hoping that when I read it to her she would recognize it and confirm that it was true. She was always asking me to read to her the stories I wrote. I do not know why. Perhaps it was because I wrote about so many different subjects. I asked her if she would like to hear a story

I had written. She said she would love to hear my story so I picked up my notebook, opened it and read.

When I finished I glanced down into her face and saw tiny tears in her eyes. With softness in her voice she said, *"Oh, Linda that was you and Poppy"*, Poppy being what she called her father. She told me all about the day that her Poppy had given me a "blessing". It was word for word as Ma had told me so many times over the years. I chuckled knowing that my mother's question to me would be about what Pa had said to me. I never told her what he said but that moment between us was precious, one that I will treasure forever. A short time later, my mother died.

Linda Martin

MESSAGE

The blessing ceremony my grandfather gave me has made me realize how much he loved me. One of the most important things he taught me was the assurance that God loves me.

SONG

Blessed Assurance, Jesus Is Mine

CHAPTER 15: *Family of God*

When I was about six years old, I was near our barn when I saw a beautiful piece of yarn on the ground. I went over to pick it up and the "yarn" moved. I bent over and looked closely at it and it opened its mouth, as if to say hello. I gently picked it up and it wrapped itself around my arm and hand. I thought it was giving me a hug.

"*Oh, how beautiful you are*", I said and decided to show my grandmother and mother my pretty new friend. I put him behind my back and walked into the kitchen where all the ladies were, my mother, grandmother and several neighbors. There they sat with their aprons filled with fresh apples. They were peeling apples to make apple pies, apple jelly and apple butter. Most of the apples were to be used in the community *"apple butter stir"*. This is where lots of apples, sugar and sometime spices, were put into a big brass kettle placed outside over a slow burning fire (The brass kettle was owned by my dad and he always had a silver dollar to put in the bottom of the kettle to keep the apple butter from burning.). The neighbors took turns stirring the apples with a big wooden paddle which looked similar to a garden hoe. They shared the apple butter when it was done. Anyway, I looked at the ladies and said proudly, *"Look at my beautiful big worm I found outside"*. I put him near my mother's face. She screamed, as did all the other ladies and apples went rolling everywhere. My grandmother yelled to my grandfather to come quickly. *"Hurry! Hurry!"*, she screamed to him.

He came running and looked at me. I showed him my new friend as it crawled up my arm with its tongue sticking out. My grandfather gently took my friend from me, led me outside and released my friend in the barn. I began to cry. Pa told me that what I had done, in picking up the snake, was dangerous. He explained to me that my new friend was not a worm but just happened to be a harmless snake. He continued to explain that there were poisonous snakes and what could have happened to me if I had picked up one of those snakes. I told him that God made all snakes so they could not be bad. His reply to me was that I was right. God does not make anything or anyone bad. We are all created to be a part of God's family but we have to learn what things in life might harm us. Sometimes we may be harmed even though someone or something may not really be trying to hurt us. I was thankful that day to have a Grandfather who took time to teach me the difference between something that was harmless and something that could be harmful.

I learned several valuable lessons that day. One was that I did not get a much deserved spanking. The most important lesson I learned was that we are all important in God's creation. We are all put here for a purpose.

MESSAGE

All of God's children are in a family, His family. My snake was not human but yet was part of God's creation. When we were serving in a smaller church we would always close our morning service by joining hands and singing the song, Family of God. I pray daily for others to come and join our family.

SONG

Family of God

CHAPTER 16: *The Divided Sky*

It was a beautiful day, a day made just for playing outside. It felt so great to be able to have the next three months free to do things I wanted to do. That would be just play, run and relax in the sun. No more school for a while.

I had gotten up late on this day just to see what it felt like. It didn't feel as everyone said it did. I had missed most of the morning by lying in bed. No more getting up late, there was too much playing to be done.

I walked down the road and found my friend Nancy. We loved to be together and sometimes we talked about boys. How silly they were. How they showed off by riding their bicycles with no feet on the pedals or hand on the handlebars. They were stupid we would say to each other. Nancy and I had a complete agreement on what we wanted in life and boys were not a part of our plans.

We had spent hours playing jump rope but then decided to stand at the fence and make faces at the boys as they went riding by on their bikes. Nancy was the first to hear the roar of something and she grabbed my arm. We were facing each other and she asked, "what was that loud noise?" It took only a moment for me to feel my ears ring. I had never in my young life heard anything like that noise.

Nancy and I looked up into the sky at the same time to see where we thought the sound was coming from. What I saw caused me to turn so fast that I left Nancy with her mouth wide open. I yelled to her that I had to get to my grandparents house quickly. I told her to hurry inside her house and hide. I glanced back at her as I ran with all my strength toward Ma and Pa's house. Nancy stood still like she was a statue, then

I knew it was true. The Bible was right and I had no time to waste. It might be too late now.

I had not had time to tell Nancy that the world was coming to an end just like the Bible said it would. I knew for a fact that God was dividing the world in two parts. One part was for the goats and one part for the sheep or was it to be divided first into Heaven and Hell? I didn't know anything except one thing for sure, that if I could be with Ma and Pa I would be saved. They wouldn't let God send me to Hell. They didn't want me to burn in a fire.

I reached the door of the house and almost knocked Pa over trying to get to the kitchen where Ma stood. Pa was good in knowing about the Bible but singing and playing the harmonica and "juice harp" was what he did best. Ma was the expert on what the Bible said and I knew she probably knew which side of the sky was the right side. I was going to follow her wherever she went. I did not want her to leave me on the left side, that was the hell side. I called for Pa to come quickly and stand with us because I did not want him to go to hell either. Ma looked at me and wanted to know what in the world was wrong with me. I told her the world was coming to an end and that we had to stick together. She laughed and asked me what made me think of such a silly thing. I told her what had happened with the sound and of seeing the sky divided by a big white line." I just knew that God was dividing the goats and sheep", I told her.

Pa put his arm around me and Ma told me not to worry that we would already be gone if indeed that had been the end of the world. We went over to the kitchen table and sat down. I sat on Pa's lap just in case she was wrong. She began telling me about the rapture and most importantly about being "saved". I felt much better, especially when she told me that I should think about accepting Christ as my Savior. I did not accept Jesus as my Savior until a few years later. There was much I needed to learn about Jesus and I wanted to make sure I understood all she was telling me.

Ma was the first person to share the plan of salvation with me. I accepted in my heart all she told me but I did not make a profession of faith at that time. It would come later or did it come at that time? I knew my life had changed. Perhaps, I was too young to understand it completely. Maybe, I thought I had to be a wise and godly woman like

No Journey Back

my grandmother and know the word of God as she did before I could accept Jesus into my heart. Whatever, it would be coming soon. Jesus was waiting patiently for me.

Oh, by the way, the great noise we heard and the white line that divided the sky were made by military jets. For some reason there were several flying together that day. At least this is the story some people in the community told me. I also learned that some of them were frightened too!

Thank you, Ma and Pa. Thank you, God.

Linda Martin

MESSAGE

When I was a child I loved looking at the sky but one day I knew I was doomed when I saw the sky being divided. It was a day that changed my life. When my grandmother presented the plan of salvation to me I believed. In my young heart I accepted Christ as my Savior. It was not until a few years later that I made a public profession of my salvation. It was that night I knew for certain, if the next sound I heard was the trumpet of God calling me home to heaven, I would be there.

SONG

When The Roll Is Called Up Yonder

CHAPTER 17: *Caught In the Act*

One Wednesday morning I received a phone call from my husband. He was in his office at church and remembered that he was supposed to ask me if I would present the children's message for the upcoming Sunday. I was always hesitant, never feeling adequate to bring a message to the children. I loved telling stories to my children but that was different from telling children stories before the whole church. I asked him about the sermon topic for Sunday and if he or the Senior Pastor would be preaching. I had not remembered who would be preaching that Sunday. The topic that he gave me reminded me of something that happened when I was in elementary school. I thought about it for a short time and decided that it would be a good story to tell to the children

I had a friend, not a close friend but one I admired. She was so very pretty and polite. Lucinda (not her real name) was a model student except for one thing. She loved to talk. She had a beautiful voice but after a while you would get tired of her talking. The teacher tried everything to get Lucinda to be quiet in class. She talked with Lucinda and explained that she was taking time away from the other students. She even put her in "time out" and had her write a hundred times, "*I will not talk in class*". It did little to stop her talking. Nothing, it seemed, could make her be quiet.

Lucinda was a competitive person and the teacher would encourage us to play games outside that involved action; especially of the mouth. Get Lucinda to yell maybe she would be too tired to talk in class. It didn't work.

One day the teacher told her that sooner or later her tongue would get her in trouble. Lucinda was opening her notebook to put in some more paper while the teacher was speaking to her. She turned to tell the student, sitting at the desk beside her, that nothing could stop her from talking. I sat behind Lucinda in class and was able to hear and observe everything that happened next. Lucinda's pencil dropped off her desk and she bent over to pick it up. Somehow, I still cannot understand how it happened but when she bent over she was still talking and the notebook suddenly closed shut. I watched in horror and amusement (sorry about that) as Lucinda began making horrible noises in her throat. The teacher ran to her and "unlocked" the notebook. Lucinda's tongue was bleeding. It did take a few days for her tongue to heal. Otherwise she was fine. Yes, the talking came under control at last. She had learned her lesson in grade school. I lost contact with her so I never knew if she still possessed the *gift of gab*.

I told this story to the children that Sunday morning with the moral that we need to watch what we say. We need to control our tongue. I told them that the Bible talks about the tongue being a two edged sword and it could hurt others. When we get a cut it sometimes hurts. When we say bad things about people it can hurt them like a real cut hurts.

I think they learned a lesson that day because they showed me their tongues and said they never knew their tongue could hurt someone.

Lucinda had taught me a lesson. I used her experience to teach my children and the children at church a valuable lesson about tongues. I have shared this lesson with my grandchildren. I remembered this lesson as I entered surgery for cancer. My voice could be lost. I thought about my tongue. Who knew exactly where the cancer had spread? God was and is good. I still have my voice and tongue. I will be careful how I use both of them, especially the tongue, because I don't want it to get caught in a trap. I will use it for God's message of salvation.

I thank God and you Lucinda for such a wonderful message for me, my generation and the generations to follow.

MESSAGE

My tongue has often gotten me into trouble but never to the point of it getting caught in the rings of a notebook, like Lucinda. Today, I am careful to guard my tongue. It is powerful and can be used to destroy or to build up. I want mine to be used for praising God.

SONG

O For A Thousand Tongues To Sing

CHAPTER 18: Santa Substitute

It was Christmas Eve in our little coal mining town and a very special time for the entire community. Our little white church was decorated from top to bottom and the biggest Christmas tree I think I had ever seen was sitting in the very front of the church. I remember distinctly that it sat on the right side of the church because the left side was the sacred place for the piano.

The women had baked cookies all week to share with everyone and the men had shopped for fresh apples, oranges, bananas and walnuts. Later in the afternoon they gathered at the church to put the fruit, candy canes and sometimes a small toy in brown paper bags. Every child that came to church that night was to receive one of the much desired bags of treats from Santa Claus. Sometimes, he had a special toy for each child. The one rule was that to receive a bag the children had to be in the play or attend the play and carol sing. I think the main attraction was definitely Santa.

It was about an hour before the play was to begin. Mother and Daddy had been busy trying to get ready for company Christmas day and Daddy kept disappearing into his "workshop" of sorts. We children had been busy running errands between Ma and Pa's house and our house. Mom was giving us a quick snack of ham biscuits and punch when we heard the sound of someone banging on our front door. Mom and Dad both ran to the door. I heard Daddy saying that he could not do it. Then I heard Mom telling him that he had to do it. I went as close as I could to the living room. I was trying to hear what had happened that caused them to raise their voices. I heard a man telling Dad that he just had to do it! Santa was sick and they did not have anyone who could be the Substitute Santa at the church tonight. Finally, Mother convinced Dad to fill in for Santa. The man must have been very confident because he pulled a Santa suit out of a bag and handed it to Daddy. He told him they would expect him at the church in less than thirty minutes. I had never seen my Dad move so fast. Mother grabbed the Santa jacket and after a long struggle Dad finally had it on. Then came the pants. Mother told him to put the Santa pants on over his regular pants. He finally was looking like Santa Claus when Mother realized he still had to put the boots on. She and three other people set to work. Two people worked on each foot. After several minutes their mission was accomplished. Daddy stood up but his pants didn't fit. He yelled for a belt. Mother yelled that he was going to be late. The neighbors were searching for Santa's hat. It was total chaos. Fully dressed, he reached for the big Santa bag, threw it over his shoulder and walked onto the porch, down the steps, onto the road. We watched as he passed a few people on the road and finally saw him turn the corner into the church. About that time a man came by our house, scratched his head and asked if he had just seen Santa Claus walking down the road!

Later that night when Dad arrived home he was exhausted but happy. I heard him tell Mom that it is not every man that gets to be Santa Claus at church and he never wanted to do it again.

When I grew older I realized it took a lot for my dad to play that role for the church and the children. He had a much more serious personality. Playing Santa at home was fine but playing Santa in public was indeed a difficult assignment for him.

I cannot imagine how the children would have felt if Santa had not been there that night to give them their bag of treats and a toy. Mother and Dad had given their time on this busy Christmas Eve to help other people. It just so happened that when Santa became sick on Christmas Eve there was a substitute for him.

There is no substitute for God. He is never sick. He never sleeps. He is always watching over us. HE IS GOD.

MESSAGE

My dad brought much joy to the children at church the night he substituted for the *original* Santa. They did not know the difference. They were just excited to receive their bags of treats and a toy. True *joy* abounded.

SONG

Joy To The World

CHAPTER 19: *The Stain*

Some years ago I was asked if I believed that I could lose my salvation. My children were in school and I wanted something to do with extra time on my hands. That was a situation I would love to have now. It was during a break in classes and a group of us were sitting around a table in the lounge drinking cokes and having a snack. Somehow the conversation turned to religion and faith. Here I was sitting with these young college students who were interested in my life. A student who was normally quiet spoke out a little louder than he usually spoke and asked me if I was sure I was *saved*. How could I know I was saved?

I told him the following story that involved my husband Phillip. We had been married only a few months and he was driving to attend college several miles away from where we lived. Phillip was traveling a mountain road to classes early one morning. On the way, he came upon an accident. He immediately stopped and got out of his car. He looked over into the trees and saw a man lying there bleeding. He went over to give assistance and comfort to the young man until emergency help came. He had seen others had stopped and were giving assistance to the young man's wife and baby.

Phillip stayed with the family until the ambulance came to take them to the hospital. After class that morning he decided to stop by the hospital to see how the family was doing. When he arrived at the hospital he was told the young man had died but the wife and baby were going to be fine. The wife had some cuts but the baby was totally unharmed.

When my husband arrived home I immediately knew something was wrong by the look on his face. He spoke with much emotion asking me if I could help him get the blood off his new coat. It scared me. I did not know if he was hurt or what had happened to him. Why did he have so much blood on his coat? Blood was everywhere. We had been saving for weeks to buy him a coat. With him going to school and working part time and me trying to work, we struggled to make ends meet.

"Honey could you please help me clean my coat? I can't get the blood off, it just won't come off," he said. I took his coat and he assured me he was fine. He cried as he told me how he had gotten the blood on his coat and about his visit to the hospital to check on the man and his family after class.

I immediately carried the cream colored coat, now stained with the young man's blood, into the bathroom. I used Clorox, lye soap, everything I could think of but nothing worked to get the blood out of the coat. We finally had to throw the coat away.

For years Phillip did not want to share his story with anyone because of his sense of helplessness in trying to save the young man's life. He tried to put his focus on the loss of the jacket but nothing helped until he realized what was bothering him most was whether this young man had accepted Christ as his savior. Somehow that morning of the accident as he and Phillip were talking, the topic of salvation had come up. Phillip did not remember which of them brought the subject up, he did remember their talk was shortened because the ambulance had arrived. The picture that stayed in his mind was one with him holding a young man in his arms on a cold winter morning beside a curvy mountain road.

The students sat mesmerized by the story I told them. I had another part of the story to tell them. It was what my grandmother told me.

I had asked her what I could have used to clean Phillip's coat that day when he came home with the blood on it. Her immediate response to me was that the man had died, hadn't he? I looked at her and asked how she knew that. She told me that *death blood* would never completely come out of anything. If the color was removed, it still left a stain. We may not be able to see all the stain but it will still be there.

I told the group that when I repented of my sins and accepted Jesus as my savior, I pictured myself kneeling before Him on the cross. I could envision Christ's blood dripping upon me, coming down into my eyes, my face, everywhere, covering me. As I stood before Him, the blood trickled down my body. Not only were my clothes stained with His blood but my body as well.

Then the whole picture hit me. The death blood of Jesus could not be washed away from me. He shed that blood and died on the cross for me, that is how I know that everyone who accepts Him as their savior cannot lose their salvation. No Clorox, washings, nothing will ever remove His shed blood from me.

I will always remember, *death blood* cannot be removed. I have been washed in the blood of the Lamb. Once covered nothing can remove it. Generations have been covered by His blood.

The students sat in silence. I sat in silence. We sat in Silence.
THE BOOD STAIN OF JESUS CANNOT BE REMOVED!
SILENCE!

MESSAGE

One day my husband came in with his new coat covered with blood. He asked me to help him clean the blood off and I tried everything but nothing took the blood out of the coat. I am glad I am covered with the blood of Jesus and it cannot be removed from me. My salvation is secure.

SONG

Are You Washed In The Blood

CHAPTER 20: *The Doll*

Many years ago on a crisp fall day I sat in the living room of Millie, a lady who was very dear to me. She would listen to my stories and sometimes tell me stories of her life. From the time I was a young girl, I loved to sit and listen to the "old people" talk about their lives. Now that I was an adult I found myself relating to many of their experiences in life. This day Millie would tell me a true story of an experience she had as a child. I was excited to know the story would be about a doll and Christmas. Millie loved Christmas and her house was the center for all holiday festivities, from Thanksgiving through New Year's Day. Every Christmas her tree was up the day after Thanksgiving and would certainly win a first prize for decorations if there had been a contest.

I sat back in my chair sipping coffee from a big brown mug. Millie had her favorite cup filled with coffee and took a sip. She asked me if I had written any new stories and I told her I had but I sure would like to hear any stories she may want to share with me today. I wanted to hear a Christmas story from her. In the years I had known her she had never shared a Christmas story with me. I mentioned that I had written a short story about Christmas.

Millie looked down into the coffee cup then turned her head and told me that she did not really like Christmas. I was shocked. How could she say such a thing? She was Miss Christmas Spirit. I surely had misunderstood. I knew she saw the look of shock on my face and began to speak softly.

She began telling me why she disliked Christmas. She told me that it was a few weeks before Christmas and she had seen a beautiful doll in the store that she wanted for Christmas. Every time she went with her parents to the store she told them how much she wanted the doll. In fact, she had told everyone she saw just how much she wanted that doll. She knew she would find it under the Christmas tree on Christmas morning.

Time passed slowly for her as she waited for Christmas Eve. Millie continued her story by saying that she had helped Mom make cookies, decorate the house and attend the special services in their little church where her father was pastor. She expressed a big sigh as she took another sip of coffee. Her first words indicated to me that she was beginning to be lost in her thoughts. She repeated that she hated Christmas. Millie told me that her father had been in town all day and she knew he was picking up her doll. Just as the sun was setting she went on with her story. Her Dad came into the house with a big box. He opened the box right before her very eyes and in the box was her beautiful doll. Her father turned to her mom and told her to please wrap the doll up in the pretty paper he had purchased. Millie wondered why he wanted to wrap the doll when he would be giving it to her the next morning.

Millie's voice dropped then became strong. Dad was taking the doll to a little girl who lived on the mountain. She and her family were very poor and it was his Christian duty to see that they would have a good Christmas.

Millie's head lowered and she was very quiet. I sat there trying to decide if she was okay. I was about to speak when she looked at me and continued with the story. Her dad took the doll and left the house. She had watched him get on his horse because there was not a road to the house where the little girl lived. He would have to travel through the woods to get to the house. Millie took a deep breath to let me know she would finish her story. She told me her hurt was tremendous. When her mom expressed concern that her dad was late and was worried about him, Mille didn't care. In fact, she would be happy if he was lost in the freezing snow and ice. Maybe he would lose the doll and the little girl would not have a doll for Christmas either.

Her voice changed again as she told of how her dad had indeed gotten lost and yes, he had lost the doll. He had prayed and God had answered his prayer in helping him find his way back home. Millie's harsh laugh interrupted the story for a second before she continued by saying that she became so angry with God. Why did He answer her dad's prayer but would not answer her prayer for the doll? She surprised me when she repeated that she blamed her mom, dad and maybe even God for her dislike of Christmas.

I knew the story was over. I didn't know what to say. I kept quiet but as all stories should this one does have a happy ending.

Several years before Millie died, she accepted Jesus as her Savior. Her life from that moment on was one of joy, happiness and a true love of Christmas.

One thing that had amazed me in all the years I had known Millie, no one had ever known just how much hate and hurt she had at Christmas time. I thank God she was finally able to celebrate the true meaning of Christmas.

Linda Martin

MESSAGE

My friend was great at hiding from everyone the anger she had carried so many years for her mom and dad. Years passed before Millie was able to release her anger and hate to the Christ of Christmas. Only then was she free to carry the title of Miss Christmas Spirit with love, peace and joy. She knew exactly what her title represented since Jesus had become her Savior.

SONG

Forgiven

CHAPTER 21: *Dyeing for the church*

Our son Randy loved to play with Lincoln logs. He had toy cars, toy horses and even toy soldiers but his very favorite were the Lincoln Logs. He loved to build buildings, big houses and forts. Even though he was only four years old, he seemed to have a talent for building things and taking them apart.

One Saturday night, he heard his dad talking about the sermon he was going to preach at church on Sunday morning. It was about building the church on a firm foundation and Jesus dying for the church and all people. While I was preparing his bath, he told me he had been thinking about what his dad had said earlier concerning the Sunday sermon. I dismissed his comments, placed his yellow rubber ducks in the tub, told him to get undressed and get into the tub. While preparing his bedtime snack, I could hear him talking to himself and the ducks. My husband was close by keeping a check on Randy or so I thought. Somehow, Randy had gotten out of the tub, retrieved his Lincoln logs and had added them to the water in the bathtub.

I finished preparing the snacks, gave a quick glance at Randy and went into his sister's bedroom to tell her to go to the den to get her bedtime snack. She closed the book she was reading, crawled off the bed and headed toward the den.

Returning to the bathroom, I reached to let the water out of the bathtub. Uncontrollable screams came out of my mouth. I was horrified! My husband and daughter came rushing into the bathroom. They saw the bright red blood colored water in the tub and froze. Suddenly, Phillip reached down and picked up Randy and we all began to laugh.

We realized what had happened. The Lincoln logs Randy had put into the tub had dyed the water bright red. I asked him why he had put the logs into the bathtub. He told us that he wanted to build a church like Dad was talking about but he guessed he did not build a good foundation. The logs kept floating away from him. Some sank to the bottom. He looked down at himself and then straight into the eyes of his dad and said, "I got dyed for church tomorrow"!

His dad just shook his head and told him that they needed to have a good talk on firm foundations and dyeing (dying) for the church!

While recalling this story, I thought about the apostle Paul and his words that we must *DIE* to self. Like Randy, there were times in my life when I didn't understand the true meaning of dying to self. God has and is still leading me on a journey that is teaching me daily what it means. From reading His Word, I have learned that it is not about me but all about Him.

I am thankful for the ways in which God teaches us these much needed lessons in life.

MESSAGE

I had experienced about everything a mom could experience in raising my children. When my four year old son decided to dye himself for the church, I knew we still had a lot of work ahead of us in teaching scripture. A few lessons might have helped him know that he should not build a church foundation in water using Lincoln logs. He is fortunate he escaped tribulation from us that night.

SONG

The Church's One Foundation

Chapter 22: *The Borrowed Tree*

It was a little before five a.m. on Christmas morning. I could hear the distant sounds from the countryside where we lived in South America. I hesitated for a few minutes before getting out of bed. I could not believe it was Christmas morning. As I made my way downstairs I could see the palm trees blowing in the warm breeze, the banana trees laden with bananas. I laughed as I thought about all of my family back in the States. They were probably envying me here in this beautiful country especially this time of year. Little did they know that I envied them for the cold, white Christmas day they would be having.

I made coffee and went into the living room to await the entrance of my children running from their bedrooms to the tree, to see what Santa had left for them during his visit that night. I curled my legs beneath me and began sipping hot coffee. Suddenly, a dam of tears broke as I looked around the apartment. I was in a strange country. My husband, children and I had arrived just a few weeks before to begin our work as missionaries. We had hopes that all our belongings would be in our apartment by now but no, they were setting on a ship in port. It would be February before everything was delivered to us. It had already been seventeen months since our furniture and other belongings had been packed and put in storage in the States. All we had with us were two suitcases each and a few footlockers. Randy was anxious to get his miniature cars and his bicycle. Angela wanted her dolls and her "Little House" book collection. Phillip and I just wanted our household to be in order again especially for this Christmas but no way was that going to happen. I wanted to cook a traditional Christmas meal and serve it on our good china but even the plates and cookware that we had in language school had been given away. We had very few things of our own.

The more I thought about all that we had given up for these long months, the more my pity party grew. I looked around the apartment and saw a borrowed sofa, chairs, the beds, everything and worse yet, a borrowed Christmas tree! I thought to have a borrowed tree was really *the pits,* horrible! Suddenly I heard a voice speaking to me. I was paralyzed with fear. How could a man get into our apartment? Where could I hide? What did he want? All we had was a few pieces of borrowed furniture, a borrowed artificial tree and a few small badly wrapped packages under the tree. Someone entering our home uninvited on Christmas Day was the last straw for me! *No way*! *I had enough*! How could he be so bold…..my thoughts were interrupted by the firm, quiet voice reminding me that I said that I wanted to follow Him, to be more like Christ. Over and over the quiet voice reminded me of my desire to please Him. Then He reminded me that Jesus was born in a borrowed stable and buried in a borrowed tomb. I began to cry softly as I realized that the one who had come into our apartment on Christmas Day was *The Holy Spirit Himself.* He had come this Christmas Day to restore the real meaning of Christmas in my heart, for me and my loved ones.

I am so thankful that the One who was laid in a borrowed manger and later a borrowed tomb now reigns as King of Kings and Lord of Lords in my life. It is the peace He gave me years ago that has served to sustain me through each day of my life, the good times and the bad.

MESSAGE

I had finally reached my destination in South America. Just for a few minutes that Christmas morning, my vision for what I was doing here in this foreign land was lost. A few words from the Holy Spirit quickly put me in my place. I replayed the song that we had sung months ago at our commissioning service by the International Mission Board. It spoke to my heart more deeply this time. No matter where I am the words inspire me and help me to see my ministry.

SONG

We've A Story To Tell

CHAPTER 23: *Miss Lucy*

Shortly after my mother died, I was sitting on the front porch of her home with one of my nieces. We were not talking because I was writing and she was lost in her thoughts as the rain came down around us. Suddenly she asked me what I was writing. I told her I was writing a story about some birds. She wanted me to read her the story. I read:

Miss Lucy hurried through the rainstorm and on to her small nest in the big oak tree. Her two young ones were constantly chirping for more food and she had gone from yard to yard searching for big juicy worms to feed them.

"I sure hope they get their fill of worms soon", Miss Lucy said to herself.

Poor Miss Lucy worked hard for several weeks feeding her young birds. One day she realized it was time for them to be on their own. She encouraged Dash and Dot, as she had named them, to try their fluffy little wings and fly from their nest in the tree.

Dash thought he could do everything, so he spread his little wings and took a running jump and **Plop,** he landed on his little behind.

"Woops", he said, *"I guess I jumped a little too hard"*. "Come on down", he yelled to Dot, *"you will love it, it's easy"*.

Dot walked to the edge of the tree branch and looked over the edge.

"No, it's too scary", she yelled to him".

"No, come on", he said, *"if I can do it you can too"*.

Miss Lucy sat hidden in the branches above them, laughing to herself.

"*Silly ones*", she said, "*Bet they will be on their own in no time*".

Dot finally got her nerve up and she took a running jump and **Plop**, she landed on her little tail feathers.

"*I did it, I did it*", she screamed to Dash.

"*I knew you could*", he said as they began jumping up and down.

"*Let's go see what else we can do*", he said.

Dot followed closely behind him as they hopped along the big road. Suddenly, there was a big roar and a rush of wind, like they had never felt, blow over them. They both tumbled into the grass.

"*What was that?*", they both said at the same time.

Miss Lucy, their lovely mother flew down beside them.

"*I guess I will have to teach you two about cars and other dangers, won't I?*", she said.

"*Oh, Mother*", they yelled, "*please teach us everything we should know so that we can be as wise as you*".

Miss Lucy held her wings out and Dot and Dash hurried next to her. They knew they both had a lot to learn and were very happy to have their mother show them how to be safe and happy little birds.

When I finished the story, I turned to my niece and we began to talk about mothers and how much they could teach us. I shared with her thoughts about my mother and how much I missed her. She was silent for a moment than began talking about how much her grandmother had meant to her.

The little birds we had seen playing across the street had taught us both a simple lesson on life. Mothers are very important in our lives. Grandmothers are very important in our lives. Together, we thanked God for giving us a great Mother and Grandmother.

The years have passed and we both still miss Mother and Grandmother. She left us a legacy of love and many good memories to share. Her love and respect for God is a special legacy she left for our family. She helped me to have love and respect for God, which continues to serve to sustain me in my journey.

MESSAGE

My niece and I learned a great lesson from Miss Lucy and her two little birds that rainy day at Mom's house. We learned that my mother, her grandmother, had taught us many lessons in life and we were grateful for her love. We praised God for creating the birds we had been watching.

SONG

All Creatures Of Our God And King

CHAPTER 24: *The Table*

My grandmother's table was sitting in the middle of my living room floor. I looked at it with the six chairs, the buffet and beautiful china cabinet and thought, I already had a beautiful dining room set that had been given to us as an unexpected gift when we left for the mission field. The members in our church had given us a big shower which had provided us with many items that we would need on the mission field. Their gifts, including money, were a tremendous blessing. After the shower, a dear friend and fellow missions worker (We had worked together in the women's mission group and girls mission group in our church.) called me and asked if we had a dining room set. I told her we did not. She mentioned that her parents (I believe she said owned) a place that made dining room furniture and she would be able to get us what we wanted. She proceeded to tell me all the different styles and colors of the furniture and asked when we would need the set. Evidently, I had not made it clear to her that we could not afford to buy the furniture because she told me she would bring me a catalog to church on Sunday and that we could choose the style we wanted. We finished talking and I hung up the phone with a heavy heart. I did not know how to tell her she was wasting her time because we were not going to be able to purchase anything. The money we had was needed to buy more important items.

Sunday came and sure enough, she came up to me and handed me the book. I took a few minutes to look through the pages. The furniture was beautiful but expensive. She told me to take the book home and look through it and let her know what we wanted. I felt so badly that she was wasting her time with us but I did as she asked and found a set that I loved.

Early Monday morning the phone rang. It was her as I expected. She asked if we had made a decision. I told her what we liked but I hesitated for a minute trying to think just how I could let her know that we were not buying anything. She continued to talk with excitement and then I thought I had caught the words that the furniture would be a gift to us from her parents. I do not remember the entire story as it happened from that point on but soon after we received a beautiful dining room table with six chairs and a china cabinet. That set served us for many years while we were on the mission field.

Now I was faced with another decision. What will I do with two dining room sets? Both of them were beautiful and both served to remind me of special memories and the role they had played in my life. I prayed.

A few days later I remembered that my brother had mentioned to me that he knew of someone who could really use some furniture. I gave him a call. He checked with the people and called me back. He told me that they were thrilled at the thought of receiving our "mission" dining room set. God had answered my prayers and a week or so later we loaded our "mission" gift on the back of their pick-up truck and watched as they drove off. Then we turned to place our new furniture in the empty dining room.

When we finished, I stepped back and began to cry. My husband was at a lost to understand why I was crying. He did not realize just how I felt with this new furniture setting in our house. I had shared with him some of the story about the dining room and why it meant so much to me. My grandmother had left it for me when she died but because we did not have the space, my mother had kept it in her home for several years. Finally, at last it was here in my home.

That night, before going upstairs to bed, I went back into to the dining room. I walked around the table gently touching it and moved back to the end where the only chair with arms sat. I pulled the chair out, sat down in it and in my mind I saw all the times I had set at that table with my grandparents, family and friends. After a few minutes I got up, gave the room another glance and there at the end of the table I knelt down on my knees. I thanked God for all His goodness and blessings that I had received throughout the years of my life. It was here, at the end of the table, next to the chair with arms, that I had first learned to pray with my grandfather.

My parents lived just a few houses from my grandparents so I spent most of my days at home. The nights were different. I spent most of them with my *Ma and Pa*. These were very special. Ma would let me wear one of her long flannel gowns and sleep on the sofa in their bedroom. Before they tucked me into my bed, Pa would tell us it was time to give God thanks for the day and took our prayer requests. He then led us into the dining room where he helped me and Ma to kneel. Then he knelt by the chair with arms and prayed.

While kneeling by the same chair in my dining room, I realized that He had passed on to me the very lifeline I would need for the rest of my life, the lifeline of prayer. It would serve to get me through all the difficulties in life that I would face, especially cancer.

Today, I still go to the end of that table near the chair with arms and kneel to pray. I give thanks to God for all his blessings especially for grandparents who taught me at an early age before I could read, how to pray. One day I will pass the dining room set on to my children along with this story on prayer. I pray that this heritage will be passed on to their children and the following generations. One generation to another generation. The journey continues.

Linda Martin

MESSAGE

My first prayers were learned at the dining room table of Ma and Pa. When we kneeled there at night, I never thought I would one day have that alter of prayer in my home. I often use it in the same way they did; sometimes for a big family dinner but mostly as an alter for prayer.

SONG

Sweet Hour Of Prayer

CHAPTER 25: *The Truth*

When another of my grandsons was born I rocked him, told him stories and on extremely rare occasions, I sang songs to him. As he grew, it did not take him long to tell me to stick to storytelling and leave the singing to someone else like his grandfather or mother. I was glad to relinquish that job to them. I did not feel the least bit hurt. I thought he was a very wise grandson and that he was going to be one of those people that could make quick and excellent choices in life.

My husband and I would visit him and his parents and when it came time for bed, I was the one to tuck him in and tell him a story. Rarely would he allow me to read a story from a book. Reading books had to be done while sitting on grandma's lap or sitting beside her. They were not for bedtime stories. I had to "make up" an original story. I was seldom allowed to tell the same one. That kept me looking around for something to use as a theme for his bedtime stories. If you are a grandparent you know what I mean.

Over a couple of years, I created stories about animals, people, trains, planes, and whatever came to mind. One night I tucked him into bed and lay down beside him. I was exhausted and hoped he would fall asleep quickly so that I could get a quick nap before my husband and I left for our home a couple of hours away. No chance of that because this night, as it always happened, he decided I had to come up with something truly unusual to talk about. I tried various themes but it was no use *UNTIL* I remembered I had seen a balloon in a Wal-Mart store that had floated to the ceiling. It was funny how many of us became engrossed with that balloon. Listening to the men talk, you would have thought the balloon was a person. They were giving each other ideas on just how they could "rescue" the poor little balloon. That gave me an idea.

I settled in beside my grandson and began my story.

One day a beautiful yellow balloon was feeling sad. He had been tied to the rack near the check-out stand for weeks now and he was tired. He had watched the children look over at him but no one wanted him. What was wrong with him? He had seen many of his friends go out the doors tied to a child's hand. Oh, how he wanted to see what was beyond the doors of the store. Yellow Balloon had talked with the other balloons about his situation but since none of them had been outside, they could not offer him any help. Day after day he stayed tied to the store rack.

One day he got his break. It was late in the evening and a lady was untying all the balloons to add more to the rack. Yellow Balloon and Green Balloon were the only two left and as luck would have it, Green Balloon was snatched up by a little boy. Yellow Balloon was all alone. Now strangers of green, blue, red and yes, yellow colored balloons were about to join him on the rack. He watched as the little boy took Green Balloon and headed for the front doors. Yellow Balloon was about to lose hope that he would ever see what lay beyond the doors. He would live forever with this group of new strangers who were tied together with him.

Without warning, Yellow Balloon began to float free from the others. He wondered what was happening to him. A crowd of people were going out the doors. He began praying for the doors to stay open but no, the doors closed. Yellow Balloon hid nearby trying to stay stuck to some cellophane wrapping near the bakery. He could not figure out how he was going to get the doors to open. He watched as others left but he was scared to leave from his hiding place. He knew the lady might catch him and he was determined not to go back to the rack again.

He kept thinking to himself and realized if he was to get out the doors, he had to have faith and go for it. He freed himself from the wrap and started toward the closed doors. The doors stayed closed but just as he floated onto a big black mat in front of the doors, they opened. Out he went. He was so excited. Free at last.

I finished this story to my grandson and he asked me questions such as if that could really happen? I told him that sure anything can happen when you have faith. It sometimes takes lots of faith but it will be worth it. Yellow Balloon had kept the faith and succeeded.

About a month later all of the family went to Wal-Mart. He and I were tired so we sat down on a bench out in the entry way of the store. As we sat there the doors suddenly opened. No one was there or so we thought. We looked up and you will never believe it, but out came Yellow Balloon all by himself. Our mouths fell open as we watched Yellow Balloon proceed to the next set of doors. Just then a man opened the doors to enter and out went Yellow Balloon. We ran from our seats and watched as he "walked" down the sidewalk and went out of sight. Later as we walked to the car, we talked about what we had seen and wondered about what had happened to Yellow Balloon. Had he made it out "alive" or had he been "popped" along the way? We were about to enter the car when we looked up and "yes", it was Yellow Balloon floating high in the sky. I personally thought I saw him smile but at least I would like to think so!

My grandson looked at me with his big blue eyes and told me that I had told the truth about Yellow Balloon. *"You just need faith"*, he told me. This was a simple statement from a young child, a statement that holds true for us all. We just need faith!

MESSAGE

Telling my grandson stories became a challenge at times but one story gave me much more than a challenge. It gave me a look at my grandson's memory. Yellow Balloon helped me and him believe that anything is possible when you have faith. My grandson reminded me of that as Yellow Balloon began his journey in the outside world.

SONG

This Is The Day

CHAPTER 26: *Beware of Job*

Happy New Year! All the celebration of Christmas and the beginning of a new year had passed and I had my heart set on a beautiful and peaceful spring. The weather was already warm and February almost gone. I had great plans for painting the house, maybe planting a garden or just taking a course in the community college nearby. I realized that I still had time to get in a few weeks of reading before I would need to begin work on a chosen project. There were lots of books I wanted to read and decided that I would look for a study on one of the books of the Bible. Big Mistake!

I looked through all my books and my husband's books but nothing seemed to be appealing to me. I knew that tomorrow my husband had his usual day off from work and since he enjoyed going out to new stores that perhaps we could go to an *everything* store. This store had lots of garden supplies, fishing equipment and lots of books, something to satisfy my husband and me. Tomorrow would be the perfect day to visit the store and hopefully find just the book I was looking for.

I was excited the next day when we arrived at the store. I saw someone taking new books out of a box and placing them onto the book table. *New books*, what more could a woman want than a fresh display of books? I already had at least a hundred books or more at home! One more could easily be added to the current number.

I quickly walked up to the display and found the religious book section. I scanned the various titles and authors of most of the books before one caught my attention. The cover was good and the topic was excellent. It was just what I was looking for to challenge me in my study, the book of Job.

I should have run away as fast as I could run and jumped into the car, squealed out of the parking lot, gone home and asked forgiveness for even thinking I could handle such a study as the book of Job. Instead I picked the book up and read the article on the back cover. I glanced through the book and felt that perhaps Job would indeed be a great challenge. I found my husband, told him I was ready to leave and handed him the book. He gave me his raised eyebrow look which told me he was questioning my choice of books but he went to the check-out and paid for the book.

The next morning when I had finished my devotional study I picked up my new book on Job. I opened it and began to read. I knew I should stop and put the book aside or maybe just give it away. But I didn't. No, perhaps God was preparing me for something great, a new adventure and I needed to be encouraged by the life of Job. I continued to read a few pages every day for a couple of weeks. Then one morning I skipped reading in the book because of a need to go to my doctor for a scheduled check up concerning a large lump on my neck that was increasing rapidly in size.

I was sitting on the examining table in the doctor's office when he told me that I needed to see a specialist concerning the lump in my neck. Suddenly the memory of the front cover of my new and latest book I had purchased appeared before me. I did not know whether to thank God for leading me to the book on Job or to fuss at Him. Of course, I thanked Him because I knew in my heart, by the way the doctor's demeanor and voice changed, that I had cancer. God knew it long before I did and was preparing me to face the many challenges that lay ahead. I gave Him thanks, that if indeed it was cancer, He would be on this *journey* with me.

If Job taught me one thing, it was that he never gave up on God. He never let the people discourage him. He stayed the whole journey with complete faith in God.

I did not know then how long or difficult my journey would be but I knew that I would not give up on God, His healing power and His comfort. He is the God of Job. He is my God. I love Him.

Beware of Job! You might be facing an unexpected journey in your life.

Be aware of Job! Through his faith in his journey he never gave up on God and God never gave up on Job. We must never give up on God and He will never give up on us.

MESSAGE

I was playing with fire when I picked up the new book on Job. I should have known that God would probably put my study of the book into action. I sometimes wished that I had chosen the book of Esther then maybe I would be a queen and have maids to do all my work. No, not really because I have learned much about what God had in store for me by reading Job.

SONG

God Will Take Care Of You

CHAPTER 27: *Uncle Raymond*

Uncle Raymond was a very special uncle and person in my life. He was my mother's brother, the only brother she had. We had always lived a short distance from each other and when he left the coalfields of Virginia and moved to another state for work, I missed him terribly. Eventually, I moved away from the area but remained in contact with him. In the later years of his life, we talked often by phone. I always made sure to call him on his birthday, special days and especially when my family or I was facing difficulties in our lives. He was the one I called first when I was diagnosed with the thyroid cancer. Like always, he had something positive to say about everyone. He was very positive in his talks with me about cancer. It's funny but I always thought of Moses when I saw Uncle Raymond. He had such a glow on his face, especially when he was talking about God.

I loved Uncle Raymond. When I received word that he had died, my heart was broken. I knew he had suffered greatly with declining health issues toward the end of his life but he never lost his love for God or his joy for life. Other than his dad, my grandfather, he was the greatest role model of influence in my life.

It broke my heart again when I realized that I would be unable to attend his funeral. I spoke with my cousins and told them that I would send a memory letter to be read by a family member. They understood and I sent a version of the following letter which was read at his *going home* service.

Uncle Raymond

I set here this morning to write a few memories of my Uncle Raymond. My mind is filled with so much that I could write a book but I will just share a few special times in my life with him over the years. Let's begin, not in any special order but as they come to me.

Last Sunday night (November 1) as I sat in church, I opened my bible to the front where I had written the date I was baptized by Uncle Raymond. The ground was covered with a deep snow, the river partly frozen but there stood Uncle Raymond in the middle of the river waiting patiently for me to be baptized. My mother looked over at me and said, "Linda, I am afraid if you go into that water you will catch pneumonia. Why don't you wait for another time?" "No" I said, "Uncle Raymond is in the water, it will be okay". You know, I never even got a *sniffle*. Uncle Raymond was there and everything was just fine. In fact he had just baptized me and my dad.

I recalled a time on a warm summer evening, Uncle Raymond, his wife and I had walked to the old school building in the hollow where we lived to attend a revival service. I was very young and didn't know much about revivals but it sounded good. During the service, I recall the preacher saying things about God, love and lost people. The next thing I knew, Uncle Raymond was on his knees up front in the old classroom. Later as we walked home, I looked up at the bright shining full moon and heard my aunt and Uncle Raymond talking about how they were now Christians. I looked at Uncle Raymond's face as he walked beside me. I knew he looked different. His face was shinning brighter than the full moon. I now know it was the glow of God upon him. Through all the years, I never saw the glow leave him.

Shortly after that night, he did a terrible thing (at least the men of our hollow said). He removed a big beautiful pool table from his house and put it in the basement. He said he thought it was wrong for him to have a pool table in his house and people using it to bet on games. People offered to buy the table from him but to my knowledge it remained in the basement molding and unused. He never compromised on his beliefs no matter what the cost was to him. His Christian values, devotion to God and his family always remained a priority to him.

I could go on and on but let me close with my thanks to Uncle Raymond for so very much he had given to me. I thank him for all his prayers and encouragement that he gave to me as I underwent surgery for stage three thyroid cancer, last year. Uncle Raymond was there for me just as he had always been my stronghold in times of joy and trouble. I thank him for being such a great and loving father to his children, to his children's children and to future generations. His name will be honored among men.

This year on his birthday there will not be a card sent to him from me but instead I think I will just have a big piece of chocolate cake and a big glass of ice cold milk. I will sit back and imagine him licking his lips and saying, "Now Lord, don't you think we could just have some chocolate cake and ice cold milk at the big banquet you are planning for all of us one day"?

Who knows what he can talk God into doing!

I love you and will miss you my dear Uncle Raymond.

Linda Martin

MESSAGE

Uncle Raymond's face glowed after he accepted Christ as his Savior. I was fascinated by the change in him. He immediately changed from the old man to a new man. God was the center of his life. If Uncle Raymond had not been in my life, I would have missed out on many blessings. One of the greatest blessings was having him baptize me in an ice cold river one Sunday in February. I am glad he decided to follow Jesus.

SONG

I Have Decided To Follow Jesus

CHAPTER 28: *Letters*

Hello my dear son and daughter-in-law,

    I wanted to write this letter to you while the special blessing event was still fresh in my mind. I really appreciate you allowing me to pass on the blessing to my granddaughter. I had prayed for some time about the special name to give my granddaughter. It is very important that her name and blessing be taken seriously. Even the choosing of the one to receive this blessing is special. I had to be certain that I had chosen the right person. How did I make the right choice? I cannot explain it in words. It was just in my heart. I knew which grandchild was to receive the blessing. I think you could see that she did accept this honor by her attention and willingness to listen. She is just a baby yet her behavior was perfect. I truly believe she knew something very special was happening to her. In the years to come, she will be able to look at the pictures and perhaps recall in her mind that special time in her life. I will continue to pray for her in her walk in life with God.

    I chose the name *Adsila,* which is Cherokee for blossom. A blossom flourishes. It is more delicate than the leaves of thorns that surround it and its beauty is always in the eye of the beholder. Adsila has already blossomed in the hearts of us and others. She, at her birth, became planted as an eternal blossom in our hearts; a beauty, a wonder, a joy and a special blessing to all who know and will know her.

    Her personality name is Snow Dove. Snow is gentle, it is strong. It can bring joy, excitement and peace. Each snowflake is like no other. It has power to bring laughter, but it can, when stacked one upon another, become powerful enough to make great changes to ones' life. It can change ugliness into things of beauty. She will, by her first name of Snow, have strength along with much gentleness.

The name Dove is the name of endearment. Again, she is and will continue to be an endearment to us.

My prayer for her, our Snow Dove is:

May your life be pure, strong and may you have a gentle heart, melting into warmth for all who know you. May you have a reliance on God with wisdom beyond your years and a remembrance of your grandmother's and great great grandfather's heritage. May you pass it on to future generations.

I cannot share with anyone what I shared with Snow Dove because this has been the custom for generations, so I have been told. If she wishes to share, when she remembers, she is free to do so. When she chooses the one for the blessing from the next generation, her words must be kept between the two of them.

Love,
Mom

Letter to Snow Dove

Each day of your life, dear Snow Dove, you will know in your heart what I said to you, your parents and your father's father on the day of your blessing. Your parents put a silver bracelet around your arm and pledged their guidance, protection and love to you. Honor them, honor God and one day when you choose the one to give this special blessing, you will feel another step of completeness in your life's journey.

May you always honor God.

Love,
Mi Mi

Linda Martin

MESSAGE

I am amazed that I could have the opportunity to pass on the blessing that my grandfather gave me many years ago. I am a blessed grandmother and dearly love all my grandchildren. My children have *done me proud*, as some of the mountain people would say. As a family we have a tie that binds us from the past generations to the new generation.

SONG

Blest Be The Tie That Binds

CHAPTER 29: *Generations Come, Generations Go*

I have written in this book of my desire to see the birth of my grandchildren and great grandchildren and to see them grow up and know and believe in God; the God that most of my family has loved, accepted and worshiped for generations. I believe that most of us will not remember the material things our loved ones have given us or their accomplishments. We will remember their words of encouragement, their gentleness, their small expressions of love especially *I love you* and most of all that they loved God. How blessed we will be, when in the passing of our generation, that we can do the same for those we love and for our God. Generations come and generations go.

She was less than an hour old when he came into the small bedroom to take her from her mother's arms. He gently lifted her pink squirming body close to his and reached for an old brown blanket lying nearby. He made his way to the porch. Carefully he wrapped her tightly to keep out any hint of snow from reaching her. Her grandmother yelled out to him to bring the baby inside. He paid no attention but sat down in the old rocking chair and lifted her up so he could see her wrinkled pink face. She opened her eyes for a few seconds as if to acknowledge that she was very content to be in his strong hands. He stood and unwrapped the blanket gently from her and stretched out his arms, lifted her up as his ancestors had done for so many years. He spoke in a whisper as the minutes passed. He put the blanket tightly around her, put her on his warm shoulder and whispered into her ear. Slowly he turned her tiny body and looked into her deep brown eyes and then her grandfather retraced his steps back into the small bedroom and lay Linda gently into her mother's arms.

Time passed and the small hand became larger but it was still not as strong as his hand had been. She reached out to the old man, his hair white as snow and many years of age upon his face. She slowly turned his face toward hers so she could look into his big brown eyes. They were now covered with a glaze but she could see beyond that and to the beauty and warmth beneath them. She gently took his worn and calloused brown hand into hers and kissed it. Tears dropped down as if to wash away the pain. She bent down closer to him and placed her head on his shoulder. She whispered softly into his ear. After a few minutes, she again looked into his eyes then turned to see a bright light coming near him. He extended his arms upward and Linda said, "one day we will be together again". She turned, retraced her steps back to the small hospital waiting room and sought strong arms to give her comfort. A great love in her life had gone to Heaven.

Many years would pass before I would be able to stand on a back porch, hold my granddaughter with outstretched arms, look deeply into her beautiful blue eyes, then put her on my shoulder and whisper into her ears the "blessing" passed to me years ago.

One generation has gone – another generation has come!

Snow Dove has come. The grandsons have come. Each will contribute of their own uniqueness to the next generation. The journey continues. No journey back.

No Journey Back

MESSAGE

Some messages can best be expressed in a simple song. My grandfather's favorite song was *I'll Fly Away*. Early one morning he did just that, right into heaven.

SONG

I'LL FLY AWAY

Appendix

Photos of Paintings

It's a warm beautiful Sunday afternoon and I have a goal before me. My goal is to submit the final pages of this book to the publishing company in the morning. I thought the manuscript was complete but I was reminded by several people that I had not mentioned two more paintings I had done. Therefore I have included black and white photos of the colored paintings along with a short explanation for each, including the first painting mentioned in chapter nine titled Finger Paints.

Photo Number 1

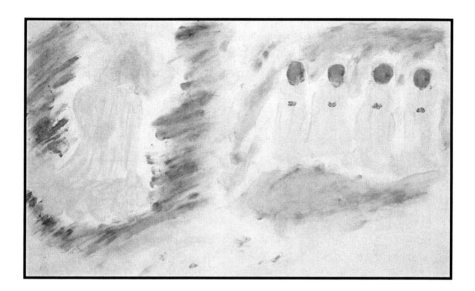

It is difficult to see the details on the robe that I referred to that were not there until the next morning. My husband and others remarked that the bottom folds of the robe appeared to have faces within it. The dark lines surrounding Him in the photo are colors in a rainbow. The four angels had deep golden hair. Their faces were all identical and were surrounded by a light golden glow. The fingers of their hands were intertwined as if they were praying. I leave each to his or her interpretation but I tried to paint this from what I remembered seeing in the operating room. I continue to thank God for this vision.

Photo Number 2

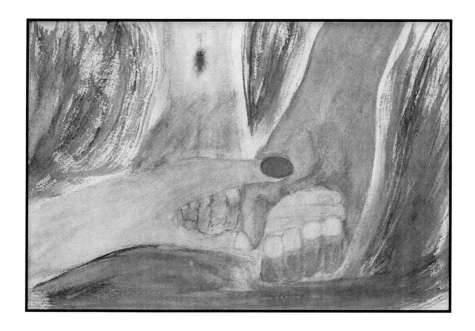

The photo of the hands is from the second picture I painted. This painting was inspired from the experience referred to in Chapter 4. Again, I felt I was being led to do this. My husband told me he would prefer to take me to purchase oil or water paints if I would be doing more paintings. I gave in to him this time and am glad I did. The painting background is sky blue. Each hand has a different shade of light to medium skin tone. For some reason, I remembered that my nails were polished a deep rose color, so I included that color on my thumb nail. I do not know why I painted the third hand with distorted fingers and a nail pierced wrist. I was really shocked when I looked at the painting later. I had been in deep thought about how much God had done for me and what Jesus had done in giving His life on the Cross, so I guess I painted as it was within my heart.

Photo Number 3

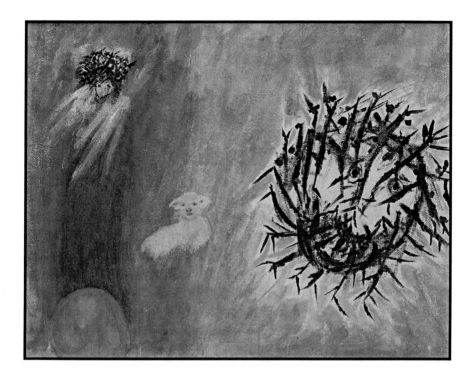

The last picture I painted began with the urge to paint a picture of Jesus which I knew would be difficult. I sat before a blank canvas for a couple of days reminding myself that I certainly did not plan to share these pictures with anyone. I only wanted to honor God and do my best. Finally, I picked up the brush and dipped it into the flesh color paint and painted a face. A feeling of unrest came into my soul while painting the eyes, nose and black hair. I stopped, looked at the picture and remarked aloud to God that I felt the picture looked too much like a woman, feeling that Jesus would look more masculine. Maybe it was a preconceived idea but it was not what I had in the picture. With the feeling of unrest still within me, I left this part of the painting and began painting a wreath of thorns on the opposite side.

After resting for an hour or so, I returned to the sunroom where I had my painting supplies and sat down to finish the image by painting the robe of Jesus with colors of greens and browns. I painted a sun or was it the moon under "his" feet and then backed away from the picture to dip my brush into white paint in order to erase everything I had done. Something was not right. While painting several strokes of white to erase the image I heard a loud *No, leave it alone*! I threw the brush down and after a few minutes turned to finish the crown of thorns. When the crown was finished, I reached to move the painting and saw eyes looking at me through the crown of thorns. I stared at the picture realizing it seemed to be a face with a mouth and beard. Then I heard the words that the painting was not finished because I had to paint a lamb between the woman and the crown of thorns (I had finally realized the painting was to be a woman). I laughed out loud because I knew that painting a lamb would be impossible. I thought about what a horrible painter I was and what was the use of me wasting my time painting these pictures (I don't think God liked that and I have since repented of those thoughts). I told my husband I had to paint a lamb and he just laughed and told me to continue to be obedient to God.

He took me to an art store but we could not find anything on how to paint a lamb. We purchased a children's book with pictures of lambs but that didn't help. I tried to paint a lamb, day after day, but it was of no use. I gave up and put the paints away deciding to forget the lamb but the image of the eyes within the crown of thorns haunted me and I began to pray. I don't know how long I prayed but I retrieved my painting supplies, picked up a brush and dipped it into the white paint. I told God that He would have to paint the lamb for me. I put the brush on the canvas and in a matter of just a few minutes there lay between the woman and the crown of thorns a beautiful white lamb. I know that I am prejudiced but that little lamb has a precious face that makes me want to reach out and pet it. God is so great!

When the picture was finally finished, the background had different shades of yellow and gold, the crown was dark brown and the woman had a wreath with jewels on her head. She is dressed in her robe of greens, browns with several large white streaks across the top of the robe. I am so thankful that God did not let me destroy what has become my favorite picture. I wish you were able to see it in living color.

About the Author

Linda Martin is a minister's wife. She and her husband have served with the International Mission Board, North American Mission Board of the Southern Baptist Convention, and the Southern Baptist Conservatives of Virginia. She has spoken in various churches and women's groups throughout Virginia. Linda grew up in the Appalachian coalfields of southwestern Virginia and currently resides in Roanoke, Virginia. She has two children and seven grand children.

CPSIA information can be obtained at www.ICGtesting.com
265199BV00002B/3/P